THE GREAT MANCHURIAN PLAGUE OF 1910–1911

The Great Manchurian Plague of 1910–1911

The Geopolitics of an Epidemic Disease

WILLIAM C. SUMMERS

Yale

UNIVERSITY PRESS

New Haven and London

Yale University Press books may be purchased in quantity for educational,
business, or promotional use. For information, please e-mail sales.press@yale
.edu (U.S. office) or sales@yaleup.co.uk (U.K. office).

Set in Janson and Monotype Van Dijck types
by Tseng Information Systems, Inc.
Printed in the United States of America.

Library of Congress Cataloging-in-Publication Data
Summers, William C.
The great Manchurian plague of 1910-1911 : the geopolitics of an epidemic
disease / William C. Summers.
p. cm.
Includes bibliographical references and index.
ISBN 978-0-300-18319-1 (alk. paper)
I. Title.
[DNLM: 1. Epidemics—history—China. 2. Epidemics—history—Russia.
3. Plague—history—China. 4. Plague—history—Russia. 5. Epidemics—
prevention & control—China. 6. Epidemics—prevention & control—Russia.
7. History, 20th Century—China. 8. History, 20th Century—Russia.
9. International Cooperation—history—China. 10. International
Cooperation—history—Russia. 11. Politics—China. 12. Politics—Russia.
WC 355]
614.4′951—dc23   2012015899

A catalogue record for this book is available from the British Library.

This paper meets the requirements of ANSI/NISO z39.48-1992 (Permanence of
Paper).

10 9 8 7 6 5 4 3 2 1

publication of this book is enabled by a grant from
Figure Foundation

Contents

Preface

The historian sees disease, especially epidemic disease, as a perturbing agent that can lead to better understanding of a particular period, culture, or social structure. We can understand different cultures and historical events by the ways nations and peoples respond to, and deal with, epidemic diseases.

Although much has been said about the Manchurian plague of 1910–1911, it remains a fruitful context to consider briefly three main features: a contextualized account of the origins and spread of plague in one of the last major episodes of the third global pandemic; the uses to which medical science put the plague; and the role of the plague in the geopolitics of the period. My goal has been to examine in some detail, but over a relatively short time span, the context of what became the "Manchurian Question," the impact and responses to the plague in specific settings in Manchuria that represent competing national interests and approaches. In particular I focus on the special role of medical knowledge in the immediate period just after the development of germ theories of disease and the discovery of the plague bacillus.

The ecology of disease is a current concept that provides my framework. Crucial events, both local and global, both technical and cultural, disrupted the ecological equilibrium in which plague existed in China. This work helps show the interrelationship of the advances in the German chemical dye industry, the world market for fur fashions, the new routes of transport and population movements, Chinese-Manchu cultural clashes, and international political rivalries, all of which contributed to the explosive plague epidemic and its attendant sixty thousand deaths.

Acknowledgments

The initial impetus for this study was the remarkable work by Carl F. Nathan, which I used in a Yale seminar on the global impact of epidemic diseases. His publications pointed the way for the elaboration of the story that is the theme of this book. Along the way I have been assisted by many colleagues, students, archivists, and friends. The following deserve special thanks: the late Frederic (Larry) Holmes, my friend, mentor, and critic as I have tried to learn the craft of the historian; Bert Hanson for alerting me to useful sources in unusual places; Boris Petrov for help with the Russian language material; librarians and archivists at the Yale Library, the Houghton Library at Harvard, the New York Academy of Medicine, and the National Archives. Thomas Hahn provided images from his exceptional collection of historical photographs. I have had helpful discussions with China specialists including Robert J. Perrins, Ruth Rogaski, Marta Hanson, Beatrice Bartlett, and Jonathan Spence, and I have enjoyed contacts and support from the family of Wu Liande as well. Mark Achtman was generous with his advice about *Yersinia* phylogenetics.

Note on Romanization of Chinese Words

Place names, when first used, are given as they appeared in the original sources or as commonly used today. The current pinyin romanization is given in parentheses if the original source is not in pinyin, so that the reader can locate them on current maps. The romanizations found in original documents, which usually approximate the Wade-Giles system, though often not exactly, are used primarily. Direct quotes retain the romanization used in the original. In a few cases, when names or terms not in Chinese are widely known in the West, for example, Port Arthur, Mukden, Harbin, they are used with a parenthetical indication of the modern Chinese name in pinyin. A similar convention is followed for personal names.

CHAPTER ONE

Plague Comes to Manchuria

"Human activity in this place seems to have completely died out; the streets are empty and deserted and all the houses are left desolate. Those who were not struck by the plague in the town itself fled terror-stricken and were overtaken by the black epidemic outside the town. The bazaars and markets are closed. Dogs alone roam in the streets, howling and feeding on the corpses of their former masters. The stench is horrible. The hospitals are abandoned. There are no ill people any more and no medical men—all have died. Only on a few beds lie the dead bodies of those who expired last."[1]

This depressing account of disease and devastation is not about Boccaccio's Florence of the fourteenth century or Defoe's London of the seventeenth century, but about a thriving commercial region of major concern to the Great Powers in the twentieth century. Beginning in October 1910, a major epidemic of pneumonic plague swept through Manchuria (fig. 1);[2] by the spring of 1911 it had killed between forty-five thousand and sixty thousand people. The plague and its aftermath were to play an important role in the geopolitical events leading up to the Japanese takeover

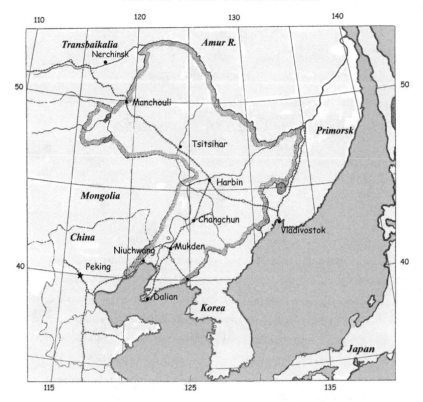

Figure 1. Manchuria in 1910. Based on a map by W. D. Turnbull, in P. H. Clyde, *International Rivalries in Manchuria, 1689–1922*, 2d ed. (Columbus: Ohio State University Press, 1928).

of Manchuria and the complex causes of World War II. The concentrated force of this epidemic, its mortality rate of nearly 100 percent, and its occurrence in a region of international competition and diplomatic struggle all contributed to the importance of and interest in the Manchurian plague. The "Manchurian Question" was of immense concern to the United States, which had just enjoyed its first taste of successful international leadership:

2

Theodore Roosevelt's brokering the peace treaty of 1905 that ended the Russo-Japanese War over territorial hegemony in Manchuria and Korea. Russia, on the other hand, was intent on retaining what it could of its centuries-old foothold in East Asia. Japan, modernizing after the Meiji Restoration in 1868, was flush with international ambition and expansionism in Korea and Manchuria, responding to its own version of Manifest Destiny. China, under the yoke of war reparations owed both to the Western powers and to Japan as a result of the disastrous Sino-Japanese War of 1894–1895 and the ill-fated Boxer uprising in 1900, was struggling with its first efforts at modernization while still governed by the decaying and increasingly ineffective Qing dynasty.

Was the Manchurian plague just another unfortunate tragedy of humankind? Or did it play a more pivotal role in history? I shall examine the particular local contexts of this epidemic: the geopolitics of national ambitions in Manchuria, the dynamics of power, and the legacies of past encounters between nations and cultures. I shall also explore the interplay between technology, history, and disease, as well as the role of railroads, agricultural markets, and the new microbiology of the nineteenth century. Furthermore, I shall consider the various "uses" of disease: as a tool of political machinations, as a vehicle to study nature and medical science, and lastly as an opportunity for fame and fortune.

First, I consider plague and its periodic pandemics to set the scene for the specific conditions, local contexts, and scientific advances that were part of the Manchurian plague of 1910–1911. I then focus attention on this great plague itself. Chapters 2, 3, and 4 will examine, in turn, the local Manchurian environment, the political conflicts, the developing technological changes in China, particularly the railroads and the burgeoning industrialization of this region of East Asia, followed in Chapter 3 by a detailed account of the epidemic itself, how it affected the three major cities, each with a different culture and background, as well as the intervening hinterlands. Chapter 4 will study the accounts of the Plague Conference in Mukden both as a window on the scientific, medical, and public health knowledge at the time, but also as an exemplar of geopolitics of the Great Powers in the Far East and the fragile Sino-Japanese balance at the twilight of the Qing dynasty and on the eve of the Japanese expansionism that, in the 1930s, led to the occupation and takeover of Northeast China by Japan under the Manchukuo regime.

With a clear picture of this specific plague before us, Chapter 5 will revisit ongoing historical controversies surrounding the biology of the plague and its origins in Northeast China and Central Asia. Finally, in Chapter 6 this great plague will be situated in the larger context of both colonial and post-colonial histories of disease, but also in the more general medical history of plague, epidemics, and national interest.

Plague is a word that conjures up fear and mystery along with images of hopelessness and social chaos. All these reactions have historical validity. Although the word has a general meaning consistent with the historical reality, since the late nineteenth or early twentieth century and the advent of germ theories of disease, the term has taken on a more specific meaning. With the identification of the microbe responsible for the cause of the disease recognized by Western medicine as "The Plague" (French: *la peste;* German: *die Pest*), most writers identify plague as the illness associated with infection with the bacterium *Yersinia pestis.* Medical historians are in general agreement that in the last two millennia there were three great, almost worldwide pandemics of plague. The first, known as the Plague of Justinian, probably arose in central Africa and then spread to the Mediterranean countries through Egypt in the sixth century. Although not all the deaths can be attributed to plague, the mortality in this pandemic has been estimated at 20–30 percent of the population.[3] The second pandemic originated in central Asia, spread to the Crimean ports in the fourteenth century, and then invaded all of North Africa and much of Europe.[4] This was the pandemic subsequently known as the "Black Death." The most recent pandemic stared in Yunnan province in China in the nineteenth century and reached Hong Kong in 1894.[5] Modern transport systems such as the steamship and the railroad promoted the spread of this outbreak to new areas and established the organism in countries previously uninfected by the plague germ.

Early medical writers such as Guy de Chauliac (1300–1368) recognized that there were two manifestations of what seemed to be the same epidemic illness: one with primarily respiratory symptoms and another with more systemic manifestations, especially swelling in the armpit and groin regions.[6] The prominence of swelling in the groin, called *bubo* in Latin, from the Greek βουβῶν (groin), gave the name to the bubonic form of plague. The illness with prominent lung symptoms was termed the pneumonic form.

Traditional explanations for these periodic epidemics recognized the contagious aspect of plague as well as its indiscriminate devastation. During the Black Death of 1348–1349, contagion was attributed to physical contact with infected individuals or their belongings, to poisons in the water supplies, and to "evil looks" from suspicious people. The causes of the plague ranged from divine retribution to rare celestial happenings and particular meteorological conditions.

Although the great pandemics were rare, there have been

regular and rather frequent local outbreaks of plague in many areas of the world. These have attracted less attention as historical events, yet they have been important in local contexts. For example, five major epidemics of bubonic plague struck northern Italy in the fourteenth century and are primarily reported in local chronicles.[7] In other places and at other times, plague has been a recurrent phenomenon as well. The famous journalist and storyteller Daniel Defoe chronicled the 1665 Plague of London in *A Journal of the Plague Year* (written as a work of fiction in 1722). Even in our own time, epidemic plague is not unknown: in 1994 there was an outbreak of what was alleged to be plague centered in the city of Surat in Gujarat state in India, with 5,150 suspected cases and 53 deaths.[8]

Our current understanding is that the same bacterium (*Yersinia pestis*) is the "causative agent" (in the sense of Robert Koch) of both the bubonic and pneumonic forms of plague. Both humans and other animals are susceptible. One form of the disease results from infection by the bite of an infected flea. Bacteria are thus introduced directly into the body at the site of the bite and are carried centrally in the lymphatic channels. They are then trapped in the regional lymph nodes, where they establish a fulminate infection with abscesses and sometimes retrograde infections.

The swollen lymph nodes, most obvious in the groin and armpits, the buboes, gave rise to the modern name of *bubonic plague*. The patient experiences the effects of systemic bacterial infection with shock, fever, and circulatory collapse. If, instead of being inoculated by the bite of a flea, one is infected by an inhaled aerosol, the primary site of infection is the lung; rapid growth of the bacteria and destruction of lung tissue produces first a bloody cough, rapid loss of lung capacity, then fever and death. This form is called *pneumonic plague*.

Plague in the bubonic form was well known in China and was often associated with an epizootic among rats prior to the appearance of the disease in humans. A widely quoted Chinese poem from the late eighteenth century describes the situation vividly:

Dead rats in the east,
    Dead rats in the west!
As if they were tigers,
    Indeed are the people scared.
A few days following the death of the rats,
    Men pass away like falling walls!
Deaths in one day are numberless,
    The hazy sun is covered by somber clouds.
While three men are walking together,
    Two drop within ten steps!
People die in the night,
    Nobody dares weep over the dead!
The coming of the demon of pestilence
    Suddenly makes the lamp dim,
Then it is blown out,
    Leaving man, ghost, and corpse in the dark room.
The crows caw incessantly,
    The dogs howl bitterly!
Man and ghost are as one,
    While the spirit is taken for a human being!
The land is filled with human bones,
    There in the fields are crops,
To be reaped by none;
    And the officials collect no tax!
I hope to ride on a fairy dragon
    To see the God and Goddess in heaven,
Begging them to spread heavenly milk,
    And make the dead come to life again.[9]

Western medicine at the end of the nineteenth century, however, was quite unfamiliar with bubonic plague. The epidemic of 1894–1895 spread from Guangdong province into Hong Kong, and Western doctors could only guess that this was the same disease that had devastated London two centuries earlier: they searched old texts and read Defoe's description of the London plague in an effort to learn more about the disease.

This was the era of "microbe hunters," and emissaries of the two great bacteriologic powers went on safari to Hong Kong in search of the fearsome germ of plague. Alexandre Émile Jean Yersin (1863-1943) came from the Pasteur Institute, and Kitasato Shibasaburo (1852-1931), a protégé of Koch, from Japan. Both were able to isolate and characterize a bacterium that was consistently associated with plague in Hong Kong.[10] Convincing evidence that inoculation of these organisms into humans could result in plague, of course, was absent. They relied on the constant association of the organism and the disease and animal inoculations to support their claim to have identified the plague germ. It may be noted that Yersin's isolate eventually was shown to be the cause of the epidemic, while many investigators believe that the organism eventually identified by Kitasato was simply a common contaminant.[11] Interestingly, this controversy and error has lingered for over a century, but Kitasato himself, in 1905, acknowledged that his isolate was not the true pathogenic organism, noting that Yersin isolated bacteria from the buboes, while Kitasato and Tanemichi Aoyama erroneously believed that the organism should be isolated from the blood of plague victims. Later, after Yersin's discovery of a different organism from the buboes, Aoyama confirmed that Yersin's isolate was, indeed, the authentic plague bacillus.[12] In spite of this clear evidence, modern writers, both historians and scientists, persist in crediting both Yersin and Kitasato as "co-discoverers."[13]

About this same time Paul-Louis Simond (1858-1947), another Pastorian, was conducting animal experiments in Asia that strongly supported the idea that rat fleas were a vector in transmission of plague, at least from rat to rat, and probably to humans.[14] Plague had evolved, conceptually, from a contagious disease to an infectious one.[15] Until the Manchurian epidemic, however, the pneumonic form was rare, and Western physicians had little experience or knowledge of this form of plague. Thus, this later epidemic supplied modern science with an opportunity for investigation as well as prevention and treatment.

Although sporadic outbreaks of bubonic plague were common in China, most were limited to a small region or a single village with several to a few hundred deaths.[16] In the fall of 1910, for example, a few cases were reported in Shanghai, which engendered intense public discussions, new regulations, and near riots. Still, it was not an epidemic.[17]

PLAGUE ALONG THE AMUR

Bubonic plague was well known to the local peoples of Transbaikalia and China bordering the Amur River.[18] Yearly outbreaks were expected by the local population. In 1901-1902, 114 deaths were reported in the Russian-controlled areas of North Manchuria, and by 1905, plague started to appear in the western regions of the Chinese Eastern Railway (CER) near the town of Ta Shih Chiao (Dashiqiao), but these outbreaks were limited and appeared self-contained. Almost as soon as the Russians undertook railway construction in this region, they encountered cases of plague. In 1898 the first reported cases were described in the Baicheng region, about 185 miles due west of Harbin.[19] The Russian plague authority D. K. Zabolotny (1866-1929), writing about plague in Manchuria, noted that in 1898-1899 there were 558 cases with 400 deaths in this region. The local missionaries claimed that the plague "came from the north" and was well known among the native populations, with yearly outbreaks expected.[20] In the winter of 1901–1902, for example, there were 114 plague deaths registered by the Russian authorities.[21] Local knowledge pointed to the tarbagan, a common burrowing rodent hunted for food and fur, as the source of these outbreaks, and some local Russian physicians began experimental investigations of plague in tarbagans.[22] For safety reasons, at first a few sick Mongolian tarbagans were sent to Russian researchers in Odessa, where it was found that they died with all the signs of plague. Later, one Dr. Chousef in Manchuria experimentally infected captive tarbagans with cultured plague bacilli and was able to demonstrate animal-to-animal transmission in the same cage. Whether this was effected by fleas as the vector or by cannibalism was uncertain from these rather limited studies.[23]

The Russian railway brought surprisingly modern and extensive medical services along with it. By the first decade of the twentieth century, Russia reported twenty medical stations with ten hospitals along the Chinese Eastern Railway, with an estimated ten to thirty beds per one thousand individuals in the population.[24]

Plagues and massive epidemics, along with wars and natural disasters, have long captured our imaginations, provoking our anxieties about causes, responses, and consequences, as well as our own vulnerabilities to future recurrences. In the Western mind, many of our most fearsome threats seem to have come from that vague and mysterious part of the world: "the East." Asiatic cholera, Hong Kong flu, Japanese encephalitis, Korean hemorrhagic fever, Ichang fever, Madura foot, and Oriental sore are names that remind us of the early Asian associations of these diseases. Plague, documented from the time of the Byzantine emperor Justinian in the sixth century, was, by contemporary accounts as well as current molecular paleopathologic investigations, believed to originate in Central Asia or China. By the fourteenth century, "the East" was taken as the unproblematic source of what came to be called the Black Death. Repeated waves of plague, or plaguelike epidemics, ravaged Europe and Asia with varying degrees of severity.

Historians divide the worldwide plagues into three epochs: the first pandemic dates from the Plague of Justinian in 541 and ends in the epidemic in North Africa and the Eastern Mediterranean in 743–750; the second began with the Black Death of 1347–1352 and lasted about three hundred years, until the Great Plague of London in 1665–1666; the third began in the mid-nineteenth century with new plague outbreaks in South, Southeast, and East Asia, a pandemic that waned by the middle of the twentieth century. This book is an account of the major plague of the third pandemic, one that rivaled or exceeded the Great Plague of London in both its mortality and social consequences.

While the Great Plague of London was famously chronicled by Defoe in his fictionalized account of London in the grip of death, panic, and social decay, the Manchurian plague in 1910–1911, which killed about the same number of people (some estimates are as high as sixty thousand), is much less well known. Three scholarly accounts of the Manchurian plague are available in the historical literature, and one key participant, Dr. Wu Lien-Teh (Wu Liande), has written a substantial autobiography.[25] The first historical work appeared in 1967 in a publication by Carl F. Nathan in the Harvard East Asia series.[26] Nathan's fine work focused on the international politics surrounding the plague in a most volatile region of Asia. In 2006 Mark Gamsa described an insider's account based on the diary of a key participant from the Manchurian city of Harbin and was thus able to supplement both Nathan's and Wu's accounts with the perspective of a Russian official faced with the task of plague control at the height of the epidemic.[27] The Wu autobiography provides an insider's view with the benefits and liabilities of hindsight. My account attempts to synthesize the political, the medical, and the cultural aspects of the Manchurian plague, to place it in the context of the great geopolitical game being played out in East Asia at the beginning of the twentieth century, and to extend the work of these earlier scholars to provide a more comprehensive and detailed analysis of this, the last major plague of the third worldwide pandemic.

PLAGUE IN CHINA

The Qing dynasty, having ruled China since the fall of the Ming in 1644, was confronted with a small but increasingly insistent group of reformers and modernizers who saw that China's aloof and isolationist policies of the past were rapidly becoming ineffective in dealing with foreign challenges. On all fronts, China was challenged to change, yet the very nature of the governing structures favored tradition, stability, and continuity. Foreign trade was limited to "treaty ports," where most of the import-export business was conducted by government-appointed agents, the so-called *hong* merchants (sometimes called *compradors* [buyers] in Portuguese, reflecting the importance of the Portuguese presence in Macau). Foreigners living in Chinese cities were confined to "concessions," that is, small bits of China that had been "conceded" to the various European powers. In the foreign concessions, the laws, customs, and way of life were those of the foreign power. The concept of "extraterritoriality" that allowed this practice was a source of deep humiliation to the Chinese reformers, who rightly saw it as an affront to Chinese national sovereignty.

Western educational, medical, and public health institutions often sprang up under the rule of extraterritoriality: foreign hospitals, for example, were established. Schools, clubs, newspapers, and even police forces existed for the benefit of individual foreign communities. It is not surprising, then, that any response to a widespread threat such as epidemic disease was met by a fragmented, politically colored, and often conflicting mélange of measures. Thus it was with the plague.

Plague, of course, was not unknown in China or even in the Manchu homeland and its borderlands. Numerous epidemics and recognized widespread disease are recorded in the Dynastic Histories, gazetteers, and other historical sources, dating from at least 243 B.C.E.[28] Carol Benedict cites the epidemic in Yunnan in Southwestern China in the 1770s as the earliest recorded account of what seems likely to be plague as it is known today.[29] This third global pandemic seems to have blossomed in Southwestern China in the mid-nineteenth century and slowly spread to Hong Kong in the Pearl River delta where it exploded in the famous epidemic of the mid-1890s.[30] This nidus of infection was carried forth from Hong Kong northeastward along the Chinese coast, eventually reaching the port city of Newchwang (Yingkou) in Manchurian territory in the early years of the twentieth century. The Hong Kong plague, too, has been seen as the origin of the San Francisco epidemic of 1900,[31] and the source of the endemic infection of the ground squirrel population in the entire western half of the United States.[32]

As well documented by Wu, Martinevskii and Mollaret, and Gamsa, plague was endemic in Transbaikalia and probably the bordering regions of Manchuria in the late 1800s and early years of the twentieth century.[33] Small outbreaks along the route of the new railroad from Moscow to the Pacific port of Vladivostok as well as the river towns on the Amur are described in various accounts of physicians, travelers, and railroad officials. These outbreaks were small, involving only a handful of local victims, self-contained and more or less accepted by the local populations as a periodic scourge of life in this rather primitive countryside. Thus, when the first cases of plague appeared in the fall of 1910, little alarm was raised.

The first report of the plague was by telegram, dated 27 October 1910. As reported in *The Lancet:* from a village near "the Manchuria Station" (Manzhouli) there were nine fatal cases on 26 October and fourteen on 27 October.[34] A month later a report to the *North-China Herald* in Shanghai from Kirin City (Jilin) in the interior of Manchuria read: "The plague has reached Harbin. Thirteen cases have been reported, all of which have been fatal. One infected house has been burnt, and the Russian Sanitary Department is taking preventive measures. So far only Chinese have suffered. The Governor of Kirin [Province] has issued orders to establish quarantine posts on the main roads from Kuanchentze [Kuancheng, district of Ch'ang ch'un] and from Harbin to Kirin. As yet little seems to have been done at Kuanchentze and Chou t'sun [unidentified] railway stations, which are the most important points."[35] Over the next few weeks more brief notes of plague deaths from Manchuria appeared in the Shanghai press. During the fall of 1910 Shanghai itself had been the locus of sporadic outbreaks of bubonic plague, the cause of much more local concern, precipitating several near riots and mass demonstrations. The concern in Shanghai over the failure of the local authorities to take a firm hand may have overshadowed the reports trickling in from Manchuria. Only in retrospect can one clearly trace the growing epidemic and its relentless progress along the rail lines and main roads leading southward toward the major port cities and Peking (Beijing).

By mid-January 1911, however, almost daily reports in the English language newspapers described the spread of the plague in North China. By 18 January 1911 "several cases" were observed at Tungchou (Tongzhou) twelve miles from Peking,[36] prompting the comment of one incredulous journalist that "the disease has penetrated the Great Wall."[37] The plague was recognized as the pneumonic form, in which infection is transmitted from person to person directly without any intermediate vector such as the fleas that fed on infected rodents. Quarantine and control of the contacts of sick individuals were the mainstays employed in the control of this disease, and these measures were applied in Manchuria with varying success and efficiency.

Manchuria in 1910 was in political turmoil: nominally Manchuria was under the sovereign control of China. However, on the ground there were authorities representing Russia and Japan as well as China. Simplistically, this situation represented the control each nation exercised over certain stretches of the railroad system recently constructed in Manchuria. The Treaty of Portsmouth (New Hampshire) of 1905 allowed each nation to station certain numbers of troops per mile of railroad for protection from "mounted bandits" as well as to provide railroad administration. Thus, when it came to organizing quarantines, control of populations of potentially infected people, and other plague control and public health measures, health workers immediately confronted tangled webs of conflicting national interests, treaty rights and incompatible administrative systems. No wonder the plague control measures seemed chaotic.

The railways in Manchuria (fig. 2) had been divided by the

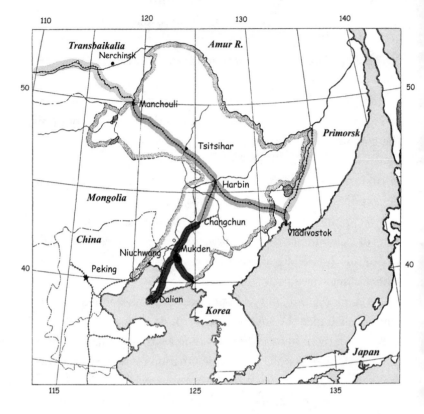

Figure 2. Railway map of Manchuria ca. 1910, showing railway control
and related "spheres of influence." The Chinese Eastern Railway (CER)
across North Manchuria and southward to Ch'ang ch'un (Changchun) was
under the control of Russia. The Japanese controlled the South Manchuria
Railway (SMR) from Ch'ang ch'un south to Dairen (Dalian, at the tip of
the Liaotung peninsula), and eastward to the Korean border at Antung.
The other main route, from Mukden to Newchwang (Niuchwang) and
Peking, was controlled by China. Based on a map by W. D. Turnbull,
in P. H. Clyde, *International Rivalries in Manchuria, 1689–1922*, 2d ed.
(Columbus: Ohio State University Press, 1928).

Treaty of Portsmouth into three sections: the Chinese Eastern Railway, running in a shortcut from west to east across Manchuria, was under the control of Russia as part of the Trans-Siberian Railway from Moscow to the Pacific port of Vladivostok. Russia also controlled a portion of the southward branch of this rail line, which extended from Harbin to Ch'ang ch'un. From Mukden (Shenyang) to Peking the railroad (called the Imperial Chinese Railway) was under the control of the Chinese government. The branch running south from Ch'ang ch'un to Mukden and on to Dalian (English: Dalny; Russian: Dal'ni, Japanese: Tairen/Dairen), the South Manchuria Railway, was controlled by the Japanese. The South Manchuria Railway also included a line from Mukden to Antung on the Korean border. Japan and Russia obtained from China the extraterritorial rights over the corridors through which their railways ran so as to maintain the railways, protect the trains from bandits, mine coal, and conduct trade along the routes. In addition to these railway guards, both Russia and Japan had substantial urban settlements along the railway and at its termini.

The main Russian presence was at Harbin (Haerbin) along the Chinese Eastern Railway. Japan developed a major port at Dalian on the coast at the mouth of the Gulf of Pechili (Bohai) at the end of the South Manchuria Railway. China maintained a parallel presence in Fuchiatien, the "Chinatown" section of Harbin, and in Mukden (where the Chinese section was called Feng t'ien). Each nation had civil and military authorities in place to administer its interests and protect its positions. The complexity of the railway administration, their paramount political importance, and their crucial role in transporting people infected with plague ensured that the railroads in Manchuria became the focus of plague control efforts as well as the main locus of contention.

Not only Japan and Russia had eyes for Manchuria. The United States, Great Britain, Germany, and France all saw this region as a rich new opportunity for economic expansion, if not for actual colonization. The promise of vast agricultural possibilities along with natural resources in coal (some of the best fields in Asia) and minerals, as well as great virgin forests, made Manchuria a new frontier for the Western powers. Even midsized towns in Manchuria had consulates representing these nations in both commercial and political activities at the local level. The various consuls were sometimes foreign businessmen who did double duty as government agents and as local entrepreneurs. They met socially, cooperated and competed in the local economy, implemented their governments' policies at the local level, and often acted together to bring pressure on local Chinese officials. The foreign consuls elected a "dean," or doyen, usually the official with the longest local service, to represent their group to the local Mandarin. The tasks of the dean often involved negotiations related to the complexities of extraterritoriality. A recurring problem that seemed ever-present was the issue of legal jurisdiction over Chinese nationals who were arrested for what were considered crimes in the foreign concessions. For the most part, it appears that Chinese were subject to foreign justice, but foreigners, no matter where they were caught, escaped Chinese justice.

One main duty of the consulates was to keep their home governments informed of local conditions. Their reports, often submitted weekly, provide rich and detailed descriptions of ongoing local happenings: trade, visitors, political unrest, and, of special interest for this study, accounts and statistics related to health and disease. Taken together, these reports from different towns and different national perspectives allow a fairly fine-grained reconstruction of the earliest notice of the plague and its relentless spread southward toward the large population centers of China.

In retrospect it seems clear that the first case of plague in the Manchurian epidemic was in the settlement called Manchouli (Manzhouli) very near the border between Manchuria and the area of Siberia then called Transbaikalia (the land beyond Lake Baikal). A death from plague was reported there on 28 October 1910 and has been taken as the index case. Soon 582 deaths were recorded in Manchouli.[38] By 8 November the disease appeared in Harbin, a Russian city in Manchuria and a main railway center, and there, too, the plague took its toll: 5,272 deaths in Harbin and its Chinese section, Fuchiatien. The disease radiated out from Harbin along with the rail lines. By 2 January 1911 it reached Mukden (2,571 deaths), and on 3 January it was in Ch'ang ch'un (3,104 deaths; fig. 3). Death was rapid and sure. The official medical records report only one survivor in 43,972 cases. The overall attack rate was calculated at about 2.25 per thousand population for the entire three eastern provinces of Manchuria. The cases, however, were almost entirely confined to the railway corridors, so the local attack rates were astounding.[39]

While the local Russian and Japanese authorities were implementing local measures, only the central Chinese government could officially act on a broad scale. In a move to respond to both Chinese and foreign pressure, the Qing court through the Ministry of Foreign Affairs (an interesting locus for public health activities) sent a young Chinese physician to Harbin to investigate the plague on its behalf. An unusual combination of circumstances at this historic moment resulted in major scientific and bureaucratic boosts for Western medicine in China. The young physician, Dr. Wu Lien-Teh, a person of talent and great political

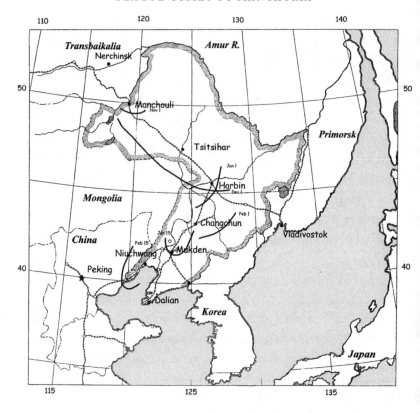

Figure 3. Spread of Plague in Manchuria, November 1910–
February 1911. Data from Richard P. Strong, ed. *Report of the International
Plague Conference Held at Mukden, April 1911* (Manila: Bureau of Printing,
1912), plate 14. Based on a map by W. D. Turnbull, in P. H. Clyde,
International Rivalries in Manchuria, 1689–1922, 2d ed.
(Columbus: Ohio State University Press, 1928).

skill and tact, was well prepared for this task by his prior education
and training.

As an astute clinician with the most up-to-date education,
Wu diagnosed the epidemic as one of the pneumonic form of
plague, while the local Russian doctors in Harbin suspected bu-

bonic plague and continued to examine patients without respiratory precautions. The Russian experts became so fixated on this diagnosis that they started a program of rat catching and dissections. Even the later diplomatic correspondence from the Russian embassy consistently referred to the epidemic as bubonic plague. A prominent French physician and head professor at the Peiyang Medical College, Dr. Girard Mesny, was sent to Harbin a little later, but he refused to accept Wu's evaluation and failed to take precautions. He died six days later. Mesny's death seems to have been a turning point, because in January 1911 the Chinese government sent troops and police to Manchuria in an attempt to control population movements and to enforce quarantines. After all, if an experienced Western physician could succumb to the plague, no one was safe. A new plague hospital was hastily set up and the old one burned down. With the ground frozen, it was impossible to bury the dead. At one point Wu reported seeing two thousand coffins in rows, with more dead on the ground because of a shortage of coffins. Worried that rats might become infected by eating the dead bodies, Wu was able to enlist the support of some local officials; then, following the traditional Chinese approach, he wrote a memorial to the throne. After three days he received an Imperial Edict allowing mass cremation of the dead bodies. This occurred on 31 January 1911.

From the time Wu arrived in Harbin, he carried out investigations on the nature of plague, the organism, and its mode of spread. His modern training in Europe led him to use approaches that were admired and accepted by European, American, and Japanese medical authorities. Probably for the first time, Western medicine was learning from a Chinese physician about modern theories of disease.

In mid-January 1911 the Chinese government asked "various

nationalities" to send experts to help investigate and treat this epidemic. The United States responded by sending Dr. Richard P. Strong and Dr. Oscar Teague, who were already stationed in the Philippines. Strong and Teague went thinking they were on a research mission, but by the time they got to China, Chinese intentions became ambiguous concerning the role of these outside experts. China was planning an international conference, and these scientists were to be invited. Meanwhile, Strong and Teague decided, with the help of their Chinese colleagues and local officials, to begin their research anyway. They conducted twenty-five autopsies in Mukden, the city where they were stationed. This number of autopsies on plague victims was far higher than had ever been done before, so Strong quickly became the world expert on the pathology of pneumonic plague.

Plague investigators, both Chinese and foreign, were interested in the source of the plague, and this hunt soon focused on the Siberian marmot or tarbagan. This animal was avidly hunted for its fur, which could be dyed to imitate sable, and was in high demand for current European and American fashions.[40] Manchurian tarbagans were in hibernation, but the few that were obtained were made available, almost exclusively, to the American researchers. Inoculation experiments indicated that tarbagans were susceptible to plague. Still, the role of the tarbagan was unclear. What was the vector? Could the tarbagan transmit the pneumonic form of the plague? These questions, it turns out, have never been definitively answered, but all available evidence supports the conclusion that the tarbagan was the original source of the plague.

In the first few months of 1911 the Chinese and Americans amassed data on pneumonic plague and were in the dominant position at the International Plague Conference, which was held in Mukden during April 1911. This conference, the first international scientific meeting held in China, evolved out of China's political balancing of the Russians and Japanese. During the epidemic, both nations proposed sending "observers" and "investigators." Japan, not surprisingly, sent mostly military people. China, reasonably enough, saw these moves as pretexts for further incursions of military units into Manchuria above that allowed for the protection of the railways under the terms of the Treaty of Portsmouth. This fear seemed to prompt the Chinese invitation to the U.S. and other governments to send experts, too. China skillfully played the American researchers against the Russian and Japanese, and soon these foreign "advisers" were converted to "delegates" to an international scientific conference. This move, of course, made it harder to include military and police personnel in what was by then being transformed into a purely scientific endeavor.

The Chinese proposal to host an international conference with the attendant prestige derived from the participation of world-famous scientists and physicians did not sit well with the Japanese. They had decisively won the Sino-Japanese War in 1895, were riding high on their program of modernization, and viewed themselves as the new leaders of a Pan-Asia movement. There was certainly an element of eugenic racial belief at work, too. Many Japanese had become enamored with theories of race improvement and saw a "whitening" of Japan in its quest for equality with the West.[41] In this context it was unacceptable for China to upstage Japan in an area of national Japanese pride, namely, modern medical science. After all, it was Baron Kitasato Shibasaburo, a protégé of the famous Robert Koch himself, to whom they gave the honors for discovery of the plague bacillus during the outbreak in Hong Kong in 1894.[42] The initial response of the Japanese, both in the public press and in the scientific community, was to boycott the proposed conference. However, as their bluff was insufficient to derail the conference planning, they subsequently, and apparently reluctantly, agreed to participate.

Young Dr. Wu Lien-Teh was the "official" president of the conference, another circumstance at which the Japanese took offense. They were especially upset that such a young Chinese should get the international prestige of such a position. By the end of the meeting, however, Wu's political skill and scientific knowledge had won the respect and acceptance of most of the delegates.

The conference lasted three weeks and included demonstrations and ongoing experiments. A tarbagan was even brought to the conference and treated as the meeting's mascot, becoming quite tame.[43]

The delegates at the conference passed forty-five resolutions as recommendations to the Chinese government. These recommendations were sensitive to Chinese positions and were not overtly politically motivated. Remarkably, the delegates, even though their individual governments (Austria-Hungary, China, France, Germany, Great Britain, Italy, Japan, Mexico, Netherlands, Russia, and the United States) sent them for obvious political reasons, were able to focus on medical and scientific matters rather well. Many of the delegates were personally acquainted or had studied with the same teachers in Europe, thus providing additional extranational relationships and loyalties.

The conference proceedings were published in Manila under Strong's editorship, and this document became the final word on pneumonic plague.[44] In perhaps one of its final official acts before the Republican Revolution in October 1911, the Imperial Chinese regime, responding to the recommendations of the conference, decreed the establishment of the North Manchurian Plague Prevention Service and recognized Western medicine as official state policy. Wu Lien-Teh did not return to the Peiyang Medical School but continued to study plague in Harbin, and in the summer of 1912 the North Manchurian Plague Prevention Service became a reality under the new Republican government. Dr. Wu trained Chinese physicians in research on epidemic diseases, and the Plague Prevention Service, later renamed the National Quarantine Service, continued until 1934 to be China's premier medical organization. Wu was recognized internationally as *the* authority and wrote a monograph in 1926 on pneumonic plague, which is still a standard reference on that disease.[45]

CHAPTER TWO

The Manchurian Question

Manchuria is a region in Northeast Asia that is traditionally the land of the Manchus, a people of the Tungus ethnolinguistic group (distinct from both Chinese and Korean), but the region has long been regarded as a dependency of China. The Chinese refer to Manchuria as the "Three Eastern Provinces" (Dong San Sheng) and often distinguish it from "China proper." It has also been called Liaotung (Liaodong), in reference to the land east of the Liao River. To the west it is bordered by Inner Mongolia, to the north by Siberia, and to the southwest it is divided from Korea by the Yalu River.

About twice the area of California, the region is a land of fertile plains, great rivers, forests, and mountains. Early Western observers compared Manchuria to the American West, with its vast resources and potential for exploitation; Europeans called it the "Ruhr of the East" and the "granary of East Asia."[1] This view, as we will see, was remarkably prescient. These three provinces have rich coal deposits and substantial timber resources as well as large agricultural regions. The climate varies from harsh in the north at the Siberian border to temperate in the south, where the ports on the Gulf of Pechili are ice-free year round, thanks to the warm southern currents flowing in from the Yellow Sea.

Located between Russian interests in Siberia and year-round ports on the Pacific rim, between China and Korea, and only a short distance by sea from Japan, Manchuria assumed new importance in the late nineteenth century and early twentieth century as trade and transportation rapidly became every nation's preoccupation.

The story of Manchuria in modern times is a story of railroads, a story of foreign markets, and a story of geopolitics on a grand scale. Into this explosive situation came death and devastation, an old scourge of mankind, the plague. Like a bomb detonator, the plague set off a chain of events that were perhaps inevitable but were certainly determined in time, place, and detail by this major medical disaster.

THE TREATY OF NERCHINSK (1689)

The modern origins of this story can be traced to the seventeenth century, when both Russia and China were extending their Central Asian frontiers along the Amur River. The Amur (Chinese: Heilongjiang, Black Dragon River) is China's third longest river, after the Yangtze and the Yellow Rivers, and the longest river in the Russian Far East. It flows generally east and southeast from the headwaters in Central Asia before turning northward to its mouth on the Tatar Strait just opposite the northern tip of Sakhalin Island. Russian settlement was driven by the lucrative fur trade, and since the region was only loosely governed from St. Petersburg, brigandage and irregular warfare were common. When Russian expeditions in the mid–seventeenth century resulted in barbarous invasions of local villages, the Chinese government sent troops, which after seven years of struggle managed to drive the Russian presence from along the Amur as far as Nerchinsk. The Russians, however, had settled the upper regions of the Amur and attempted to collect tribute from the native tribes. These tribes appealed to Peking for help and eventually, on 2 August 1689, representatives of Russia and China met near Nerchinsk to conclude a treaty that established boundaries and checked the Russian advance into Central Asia. The Chinese were supported in their negotiations by a delegation of Jesuits from Peking, and by the presence of ten thousand Chinese troops. The Treaty of Nerchinsk, the first concluded by China with a Western power, was signed on 27 August 1689 and formed the basis of Sino-Russian relations in Central Asia for 150 years. Interestingly, the four official texts of this treaty (in Latin, Chinese, Russian, and French) all differ in their language, clarity, and vagueness.[2] Neither Russia nor China attempted to exploit the potential of this region, nor did they attempt to establish much in the way of permanent governmental structures and settlements that would have exposed the weaknesses in the Treaty of Nerchinsk. Russian interest was mainly focused on the fur trade, and Chinese interest was in maintaining a secure northern frontier. Only in the nineteenth century, with its rampant colonialism, nationalism, and mercantilism, was the Treaty of Nerchinsk revisited.

THE TREATY OF PEKING (1860)

For some time, Russian opinion was divided on whether the Treaty of Nerchinsk had been a major blunder of Russian diplomacy, and in 1846 Tsar Nicholas I ordered that the whole question of the Amur River territory be reopened. The next year he appointed Nicholas Muravieff, later known as Muravieff Amursky, as governor of Eastern Siberia. Muravieff has been generally regarded as a person of capacity and vision. His task was to consolidate the Russian position in East Asia and to establish a Russian naval base on the Pacific. In 1853, under Russian imperial sanction, Muravieff occupied Sakhalin Island and thus set in motion events that would resonate well into the twentieth century.[3]

Sakhalin Island is geologically part of the chain of Japanese islands and separated from Hokkaido by only a few miles of water. At this same time, Muravieff approached the Chinese emperor to offer Russian protection against the increasing power of England in the Far East. This strategy was both logical and timely: Russia was at war with England and France in the Crimea, which provided a Russian pretext for expeditions down the Amur River to protect Russian interests in the Pacific. The Chinese, internally weakened by the Taiping rebellion (1851–1864),[4] and externally weakened by the Opium Wars (1839–1842 and 1856–1860) with England and France, were in no position to reject Russian proposals for new privileges along the Amur.[5] Muravieff, on his part, was careful to avoid unnecessary conflicts with the Chinese, and on 16 May 1856 a new treaty between Russia and China was concluded at the Central Asian town of Aigun. The Aigun Convention provided Russia with clear possession of all territory north of the Amur as well as joint control of the region surrounding the future site of Vladivostok. On 20 July 1860 Russia occupied the site of Vladivostok, its choice for its Pacific port city. With the French and British Allied Armies advancing on Peking and the Chinese Imperial Court in flight during the Opium Wars, the Russian ambassador offered the Chinese a way out: cede the eastern maritime province of Primorsk to Russia in exchange for Russian intervention with Britain and France to cease hostilities in China. Prince Kung, then in charge of the Chinese government, agreed to trade this bit of barren northeastern seacoast to Russia in exchange for its protection from the predations of France and England.[6] Both sides delivered on their promises; General Ignatieff, the Russian ambassador, made representations to Lord Elgin and Baron Gros, the commanders of the Allied Armies in China, which led to the Treaty of Tientsin, ending the first part of the Second Opium War in June 1858, and China and Russia signed the Treaty of Peking in November 1860 in which Russia acquired its long-sought outlet to the Pacific. The Treaty of Peking was to play important symbolic roles in Sino-Russian relations in the early twentieth century as well as in Sino-Soviet relations in the mid–twentieth century. Russia emerged as the historical protector of China against the incursions of the European powers.

RAILWAYS IN MANCHURIA

Important as rivers were for transportation, as elsewhere it was the railroad that was crucial to the economic and political development of Manchuria. In January 1896 Alexander Hosie, an American missionary, made a business trip from the Manchurian town of Newchwang (Niuzhuang) to the town of Kirin (Jilin), which he vividly described in his journal.[7] The journey of about 375 miles took thirteen days by horse cart with a caravan of ten people, four carts, twelve mules, and three ponies. The temperature often reached minus 34 degrees Fahrenheit. Amazingly, only fifteen years later, the same route could be traversed by train in about one day in relative comfort, with regularly scheduled passenger train service from Port Arthur (Lüshun) on the Yellow Sea all the way through to Moscow.

Railway construction in Manchuria started in earnest in 1897 with the building of the first segments of the Chinese Eastern

Railway by Russia, aimed at linking Transbaikalia with the Pacific Ocean. After much delay because of difficult working conditions, poor administration, corruption, and shortages of skilled workers, this east–west line was completed in 1903.[8] Right after the Russo-Japanese War, in 1906, Japan organized the South Manchuria Railway Company to develop railways in its so-called Leased Territories in the Liaotung peninsula. The South Manchuria Railway was under the control of the brilliant Japanese polymath Gotō Shinpei, and the entire project was the centerpiece of Japan's colonial strategy in Manchuria.[9] Indeed, the diplomatic and geopolitical importance of the railways was widely recognized. In the words of the British Foreign Office Annual Report for 1909: "Since Japan and China in the summer of 1909 settled the eight principal outstanding questions between them, it may be said that the history of Sino-Japanese relations is practically synonymous with this history of railway proposals in Manchuria."[10] Manchuria was the focus of railway development from the Chinese side, too. By 1910 there were 5,404 miles of railway actually operational in China, of which nearly half, 2,433 miles, were in Manchuria. Two-thirds of these Manchurian railways were, however, under Japanese or Russian control.[11] These railways were called the Manchurian System, although they were anything but systematic: while most of the lines were built to the British standard width of 4 feet 8 1/2 inches, some lines were of the Russian standard of 5 feet, some were 1 meter (39.4 inches), and still others were 30 inches.[12]

POLITICAL DISINTEGRATION BEFORE THE PLAGUE

Railroads in Manchuria were intimately connected to the spoils of war as well. Two wars, in fact. In 1894 the Chinese assumption of nominal suzerainty over Korea, first established by the Manchus in 1637, was challenged directly by a Japanese treaty recognizing Korea as a fully independent state, a challenge that was forcibly resisted by China. The ensuing armed conflict spilled over from Korea into Manchuria, and to almost everyone's surprise, the Chinese armies were no match for the recently modernized Japanese forces. The humiliating defeat of the Chinese by a people they often derisively called the "Eastern Dwarfs" or "Eastern Pirates" added to the sense of despondency, crisis, and need for reform in China. The Sino-Japanese War, fought mainly in Korea and Manchuria, ended in 1895 with treaty negotiations in the Japanese city of Shimonoseki.

The initial conditions of the famous or infamous Treaty of Shimonoseki forced China to cede a large portion of southern Manchuria to Japan, unconditionally and in perpetuity. This Japanese foothold on the mainland of East Asia threatened the interests of Russia, France, and Germany, each in its own way.[13] In a combined effort of these governments (sometimes called the "Triple Intervention"), later joined by Spain, these European powers pressured Japan, "in a spirit of cordial friendship,"[14] to accept a "convention of retrocession" in which its strong territorial claims in Manchuria were relinquished, but which included Japanese acquisition of Taiwan and the Pescadores islands as well as reparations that exceeded by threefold the total annual income of the Chinese government. The indemnities that Japan extracted from China in these negotiations were punishing, and in the view of some historians, these payments, coupled with additional indemnities following the Boxer uprising and interest on massive foreign loans, crippled Chinese growth and modernization for the entire twentieth century and at the same time allowed Japan to stabilize its currency and adopt the gold standard in 1897.[15]

Russian diplomatic involvement in the Sino-Japanese War of 1894–1895 was driven by its newly formulated Pacific Rim strategy, based on construction of a Trans-Siberian Railway. Shallow waters and constant silting made river travel in Central and East Asia unreliable at best, so any long-term Russian development in that part of the world required railway construction. This realization, together with a vision for Russian presence on the Pacific, gradually evolved in St. Petersburg in the 1880s, driven by an able financier and court official, Sergei Witte. Tsar Alexander III appointed his son, the future tsar Nicholas II, as head of the Siberian Railway Committee as an indication of the importance of this issue in Russian official circles. In 1891 Russia started construction of a Trans-Siberian Railway aimed eventually at the already secure port of Vladivostok on the Pacific Ocean. By the time of the Sino-Japanese War, Russia had extended the railroad to the Central Asian region known as Transbaikalia (beyond Lake Baikal). Its route from there to Vladivostok was still uncertain. Witte proposed taking the shorter, straight-line route across Manchuria rather than building a large diversion north of the Amur River, but this would require concessions from China. The Russian diplomatic effort on behalf of China to extract the convention of retrocession from Japan afforded a most timely and justifiable pretext for Russia to bring up the trans-Manchurian route for its railway across Asia.

One consequence of Russian expansionism in the Far East was the desire for railway access to both Vladivostok and an all-season seaport farther south on the Pacific coast. In August 1895 an expedition of Russian surveyors entered Manchuria to explore railway routes in the region. This was done without consultation or with little knowledge of the Chinese authorities. In October, however, Russia requested permission from China for such survey parties, and after several months of negotiation, in December 1895, the Qing court, realizing that it could not afford to build the railway itself, acquiesced. By the end of December the survey report, clearly already done by the earlier Russian teams, marked out the proposed routes for the Chinese Eastern Railway to run east–west to Vladivostok, as well as a southern branch to reach Port Arthur, adjacent to Dairen on the Gulf of Pechili.

Thus, in 1896, China and Russia signed what came to be known as the "secret accord of 1896." This agreement, not made public until 1910, ceded to Russia a strip of land across Manchuria upon which to build its railway and within which it had complete sovereignty and authority, and it established provisions for mutual defense directed against Japan.[16] By September 1896 China and Russia concluded an agreement outlining the railway project. This agreement was a vague contract for the construction of the Chinese Eastern Railway by a joint Russo-Chinese company that had virtually unlimited authority to administer an undefined area in the vicinity of the line and to exploit the natural riches in the area. The railways were to revert automatically to Chinese government ownership after eighty years or by purchase after thirty-six years. In August 1897, with much fanfare, construction started. Construction was slow and difficult, however, plagued by hard working conditions, poor administration, corruption, graft, and, probably most important, a dire shortage of skilled workers. Nonetheless, by 1900 the east–west portion of the railway was functional, and in 1903 the project was completed. Suddenly, transportation, economy, and culture in Manchuria were undergoing wrenching changes. Clearly the Chinese realized that the Russians now had direct routes not only for trade in Manchuria, but, more important, they had smooth access militarily as well. As Michael Hunt noted, "No where else in China did the railway have as dramatic an impact as in Manchuria."[17] From start to finish, however, the Russians were clearly in charge of what was only a nominal joint venture. As an example of Russia's dominance in this project, the railways were built to the standard Russian gauge of 5 feet rather than the standard Chinese and Korean width of 4 feet 8 1/2 inches.

Perhaps the outstanding icon of Russian presence in China was the city of Harbin, located midway between the Mongolian border and the port of Vladivostok. Russian surveyors for the Chinese Eastern Railway came upon a Chinese fishing village of about six houses and a nearby distillery along the Sungari River identified as Khaabin on their maps in 1895.[18] Sometime between 1897 and 1898 this group decided to base their operations for the construction of the railway in this location and started construction of what became the largest foreign settlement in China by 1910. Harbin became a truly Russian city. Its architecture from the start featured the classical as well as art nouveau styles that were in vogue in Imperial Russia at the time; 95 percent of the land in the city was owned by the Russian-controlled railway company.[19] The population rapidly increased: from twelve thousand in 1901 to sixty thousand by October 1903.[20] In 1910 the foreign population alone was reported as forty-four thousand Indo-Europeans.[21] As the main city along the Chinese Eastern Railway, Harbin was destined to become the first city to feel the power of the plague, and the first bulwark in the defense against its spread outward from its initial focus on the Manchurian border.

The railways, however, were not the only instrument of geopolitical focus. In November 1897 Germany, desiring to secure a naval base in China, seized the Chinese port city of Kiaochow (Jiaozhou) in Shandong province. Because prior Sino-Russian agreements gave Russia the rights to use Kiaochow harbor, China appealed to Russia for help in expelling the Germans. Unbeknownst to the Chinese, however, Germany had received prior assurances of Russian acquiescence to their seizure of Kiaochow. Some of the Russian Far East experts, notably the foreign minister, Count Muravieff, suggested that the time was auspicious for Russia to obtain a Chinese port city of its own, specifically Port Arthur (Lüshun) or nearby Dalian. This action was opposed by Witte, who saw such precipitous action as undermining his careful efforts to maintain cordial relations with the Chinese with respect to the Trans-Siberian Railway project across Manchuria.

In St. Petersburg, Tsar Nicholas II received a report from Muravieff, later found to be false, that British ships were in the North China Sea and would take Port Arthur if the Russians did not. Acting on this report, the tsar ordered the occupation of Port Arthur and Dalian in December 1897. After negotiations tainted with scandal and bribery, China and Russia signed an agreement in March 1898 providing Russia with a twenty-five-year lease of Port Arthur.[22] Russia also secured rights to build a southern branch line of the Chinese Eastern Railway, as the Manchurian portion of the Trans-Siberian Railway was called, to Dalian and Port Arthur. Significantly, Russia affirmed that Chinese consent for the construction of this railway "shall never, under any form, serve as a pretext for the seizure of Chinese territory or for an encroachment on the sovereign rights of China."[23] This issue was to surface again in 1910 with respect to plague control measures in Manchuria. The original agreement was refined in several subsequent protocols signed in May and July 1898, one of which set up the Southern Manchuria branch of the Chinese Eastern Railway, with Russian control over various activities along the route of the railway. Significantly, Russia, through the Chinese

Eastern Railway Company, gained control of the customs operations at the international port of Dalian. In fact, Russia decided to make Dalian a free commercial port, and no Chinese customs were established in the leased territory while it was under Russian administration.

Other national interests were involved in Russia's aggressive Manchurian policies. While France and Germany offered no objections, Great Britain saw itself being left out and sought to establish rights to certain Chinese ports to "maintain the balance of power in the Gulf of Pechili (Bohai), which is menaced by Russia's occupation of Port Arthur."[24] Japan was remarkably restrained and pragmatic in its reaction. This was attributed to its hope that once Russia had acquired its ice-free port on the Pacific, it would cease its interference with Japan's paramount interests in Korea.

While Port Arthur was viewed by the Russians as their long-sought ice-free naval base on the Pacific, the demands of the international community for a commercial port in Manchuria led Russia to develop nearby Dalian as a major commercial city, a counterpart to the militarized Port Arthur. In 1898 Dalian was a small fishing village, but soon Russian, and later Japanese, planning and construction led to its development as "one of the finest cities in the Orient."[25]

The period after the German seizure of Kiaochow and Ch'ing tao (Qingdao) in 1897 was a difficult one for China. The scramble by the Western powers for bits of China led to complex and often contradictory actions on both sides. The reactionary government in Peking, under the Empress Dowager of the Qing dynasty (the dynasty in power since 1644), was corrupt as well as ineffectual. Foreign affairs were entrusted to a few relatively low-level officials, a few of whom, for example Li Hung-chang, were remarkably skilled. In 1900 an uprising of a Chinese sect, known as the Boxers, spread from its origin in Shantung to the region around Peking and Tientsin (Tianjin). This was a violently xenophobic movement that attempted to expel all foreigners from China. Their efforts were supported by the Imperial Court (but opposed by the provincial warlords), and in June 1900 China declared war on the foreign powers. Between June and August 1900 an allied force of Germany, France, Great Britain, Japan, Russia, and the United States recaptured Tientsin and marched onward to Peking, which was sacked in mid-August 1900. The consequences of these events were perhaps not overstated by a prescient Henry Adams: "The drama acted at Peking, in the summer of 1900, was in the eyes of a student, the most serious that could be offered for study, since it brought him suddenly to the inevitable struggle for control of China, which, in his view, must decide the control of the world; yet, as a money value, the fall of China was chiefly studied in Paris and London as a calamity to Chinese porcelain. The value of a Ming vase was more serious than universal war."[26]

The Boxer uprising provided the pretext for additional Russian expansion in Manchuria. Under the general rubric of "restoring order and stabilization" Russia annexed the right (Chinese) bank of the Amur River on the very day the allies marched into Peking. In short order Russian forces occupied the important Manchurian cities of Newchwang and Harbin. Another major city, Mukden, was brought under joint Russian and Chinese administration. By 1901 Manchuria was no longer a Russian "sphere of influence" but had become an occupied territory.

THE AMERICAN ROLE: "THE OPEN DOOR"

The de facto occupation of Manchuria by Russia was of great concern to the other powers, and each was concerned that the others might gain territorial advantage through secret diplomacy with China or Russia. As in previous crises, the mutual suspicions of the powers saved China from dismemberment.[27] Great Britain was especially concerned with Russian moves in Manchuria, and it organized the support of the other nations so that China was able to put an end to the Boxer uprising without official recognition of Russian hegemony in Manchuria. The U.S. secretary of state, John Hay, was the author of the Open Door Policy, which strove to maintain parity between all the competing nations in their relations with China. This policy was implemented by joint acceptance of Hay's note of 1899, which urged the powers to follow the United States in declaring that their respective interests in China would maintain an "open door" toward all other foreign nations. Hay's note was sufficiently vague that it could be equivocally accepted by the involved powers.[28] By 1902, however, with the signing of a separate Anglo-Japanese agreement, which had the effect of recognizing "special" spheres of influence in China, Hay's Open Door Policy was in shambles. Again, from the view of Hay's friend Adams: "Hay had reached the summit of his career, and saw himself on the edge of wreck. Committed to the task of keeping China 'open,' he saw China about to be shut. Almost alone in the world, he represented the 'open door,' and could not escape being crushed by it."[29] As Adams notes, luck was with Hay for a few more years, however. European intrigue allowed Hay to maintain some appearance of common policy toward China. In the spring of 1903 "Russia held Europe and America in her grasp, and Cassini [the Russian ambassador to Washington] held Hay in

his. The Siberian Railway offered checkmate to all possible opposition. Japan must make the best terms she could; England must
go on receding; America and Germany would look on at the ava-
lanche. The wall of Russian inertia that barred Europe across the
Baltic, would bar America across the Pacific; and Hay's policy
of the open door would infallibly [*sic*] fail."[30] Small wonder that
American attention was focused on the "Manchurian Question"
and the Siberian Railway in particular.

Backed by the strength of the Anglo-Japanese alliance, and
by its drive for commercial expansion in Korea and Manchuria,
Japan first sought assurances from Russia with respect to these
two regions, and when diplomatic efforts failed, Japan directly
tested the "open door" in Manchuria by a surprise naval attack
on Port Arthur on 8 February 1904. War was declared on February 10. The outcome of the so-called Russo-Japanese War is
well known. To the surprise of just about everyone, Japan emerged
as the decisive victor, crushing the vaunted armies of the Imperial
Tsar of Russia.

The ending of this war was to involve the United States in its
first major international diplomatic triumph and marked its emergence onto the world stage as a key force to be reckoned with.
This signaled America's diplomatic coming of age, so to speak.
With Secretary Hay terminally ill, President Theodore Roosevelt was personally conducting American foreign policy in 1904.
He was concerned to maintain the balance of power in East Asia
as well as to support Chinese control in Manchuria. For the first
year of the war, each side thought it held the winning position, but
by 1905, after Japan decisively defeated the Russians in several key
battles, and with Tsar Nicholas II concerned that continuation of
an unpopular war might lead to revolution and overthrow of his
government, in early June 1905 both sides agreed to Roosevelt's

offer of mediation. Portsmouth, New Hampshire, was selected by Roosevelt as the site for the negotiations, partly for the logistical reason that it was near one end of the transatlantic telegraph cable, and partly because Washington was unbearably hot in August when the talks were scheduled to start.

The Treaty of Portsmouth was negotiated by Sergei Witte, ironically one of the senior Russian statesman resolutely opposed to the war from the beginning, as well as the architect of the Trans-Siberian Railway enterprise, and by Jutaro Komura, the Japanese foreign minister and a graduate of Harvard Law School. Roosevelt, who would be awarded the Nobel Peace Prize in 1906 for his work in mediating these negotiations, was represented at the conference by Herbert H. D. Pierce, third assistant secretary of state (fig. 4). The terms of the Treaty of Portsmouth were agreed upon by the end of August 1905 but were amended by several subarticles a few months later. Key provisions of the treaty 1) transferred the Russian lease to the tip of the Liaotung peninsula to Japan; 2) allowed Japan free rein in Korea; 3) relinquished to China all occupied territory except the leased territories on the Liaotung peninsula, Port Arthur, and Dalian; 4) restored to Japan the control of the southern half of Sakhalin Island. Several articles of the Treaty of Portsmouth deal specifically with railroads in Manchuria: Japan gained control of the Southern Manchuria Railway (Ch'ang ch'un to Port Arthur), and in article 7 the two parties agreed to "exploit their respective railways in Manchuria exclusively for commercial and industrial purposes and nowise for strategic purposes. It is understood that this restriction does not apply to the railway in the territory affected by the lease of the Liaotung Peninsula" (fig. 5).[31]

This article would become a crucial factor in both Japanese and Russian responses to the plague in 1910. This article, along with one asserting the principles of equal treatment and of most

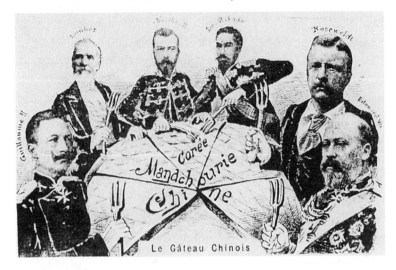

Figure 4. French postcard titled "The Chinese Cake," caricaturing the outcome of the Portsmouth Peace Conference in 1905. *From left:* Emperor William II of Germany; Émile Loubet, president of the French Republic; Nicholas II, czar of Russia; Emperor Meiji of Japan; Theodore Roosevelt, president of the United States; and King Edward VII of the United Kingdom.

favored nation status, became the basis of future commercial polices in Manchuria. Significantly, subarticle 3 specified limits (fifteen guards per kilometer) on the number of railway guards permitted to protect the belligerents' respective railway lines in Manchuria. Clearly, the parties recognized the potential use of railway guards as a cover for future military buildups.

JAPANESE POLICIES IN MANCHURIA

From the start, Japan recognized that the railways could be key to its long-term influence in Manchuria. In several ways, Japanese strategies in Manchuria had been rehearsed by the Japanese

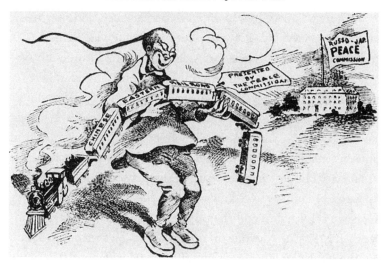

Figure 5. Political cartoon showing the "spoils" of peace in terms of Chinese control of the Chinese Eastern Railway. (From *The Evening Press*, Detroit, August 1905; reprinted in *Harper's Bazaar*)

administration of Taiwan since its takeover from China after the Sino-Japanese War and the Treaty of Shimonoseki in 1895. For one, the talented and remarkable Gotō Shinpei (1857–1929), the former chief of the Civil Affairs Bureau in Taiwan, became the de facto architect of the Japanese presence in Manchuria. As the main deputy to General Kodama Gentarō, the Japanese governor-general in Taiwan, Gotō developed theories and approaches to colonization that he would repeat in Manchuria.[32] These strategies rested on two basic principles. First was a respect for native customs and government traditions, and second was aggressive development and promotion of modern infrastructures such as railroad construction, steamship lines, postal and telegraph services, hospitals, school, and roads. He was also an advocate for effective and honest police administration.

Gotō was educated as a physician in Japan and Germany, and at the early age of twenty-two was made vice principal of the medical school attached to Aichi Prefectural Hospital in Nagoya. He was an active reformer in Japanese medical education and health care and was known for his vocal advocacy of better public health measures in Japan. A chance encounter in which he ministered to a key Japanese politician who was wounded in an assassination attempt led to his rapid rise in the Japanese bureaucracy. His activism and enthusiasm led some to call him the "proposal maniac."[33] Gotō was deeply impressed by progressive German scholarship and the power of "research" to solve problems. By 1895 he was put in charge of the quarantine program for the returning Japanese Army after the Sino-Japanese War. He brilliantly managed a serious cholera outbreak in June 1895 using the new bacteriological knowledge and was given a personal audience with the Japanese emperor to report on his work.

With the railways in the south of Manchuria as one of the spoils of the Russo-Japanese War, Japan sought ways to exploit this major asset. A major railway issue was the matter of civilian or military control. Gotō had actively promoted a civilian plan to exploit the Manchurian railways to monopolize Asian trade with the European countries and thereby gain control of Manchurian agriculture. His idea, though not original, coincided with that of his mentor, General Kodama, who had drawn up a plan for administration of Manchuria just before the signing of the Treaty of Portsmouth: "The most essential post-war policy in Manchuria is to carry out numerous secret projects under the pretext of running a railway company. The South Manchuria Railway Company must pretend that it has nothing to do with politics or the military."[34] Kodama was appointed head of the Manchurian exploitation committee in January 1906 and in July he became chair of the South Manchuria Railway foundation committee. Upon Kodama's sudden death, Gotō accepted the presidency of the South Manchuria Railway on 31 July 1906 and immediately undertook an active campaign to implement "military preparedness in civil garb."[35] Itō Takeo recorded Gotō's words on this subject:

> In short, colonial policy is military preparedness in civil garb; it is carrying out the hegemon's strategies under the flag of the kingly way. Such a colonial policy is inescapable in our time. What facilities, then, are necessary to see it through?
>
> We have to implement a cultural invasion with a Central Laboratory, popular education for the resident populace, and forge other academic and economic links. Invasion may not be an agreeable expression, but [language] aside we can generally call our policy of invasion in civil garb. . . . Certain scholars have said that the secret of administration is to take advantage of the people's weaknesses . . . insofar as the secret to administration does hang on the weak points of mankind's way of life and in fact has throughout history, it is that much more so with colonial policy.[36]

The Japanese cultural invasion of Manchuria began in earnest when Gotō established the Research Office (later the Research Section) of the South Manchuria Railway in Dairen (the name was changed to the Japanese form from the Chinese Dalian) and Tokyo in January 1908. Its mandate was to undertake research on topics as diverse as old customs of Manchuria, Manchurian and Korean history and geography, and economic conditions in Manchuria, all with an eye toward eventual usefulness in the colonial project. Gotō also emphasized the practical: he published instructions for the South Manchuria Railway employees on how to treat native customers politely, as well as pamphlets on how to manage health affairs and sanitation in his employees' homes. Most important, he undertook a campaign of major construction and modification of the railways and the public works under his administration.[37]

Modeled on prior Russian strategies, the South Manchuria Railway undertook the construction of hospitals and clinics in the urban areas along the railway zone. By 1916 there were fourteen hospitals maintained by the South Manchuria Railway. These medical facilities provided care for both the foreign residents as well as the native population. Gotō's pet project was the founding of a medical school in Manchuria, a joint venture between the Japanese and Chinese governments. The school in Mukden, Minami Manshū Igakudō (South Manchuria Medical School) opened in 1911, and as Gotō later said, it served to spread Japanese influence throughout South Manchuria and thus furthered his concept of "military preparedness behind cultural projects."[38]

Because the Russo-Japanese agreements at Portsmouth completely ignored nominal Chinese sovereignty in Manchuria, one of the political niceties to be resolved was Sino-Japanese administration of the South Manchuria Railway. By the summer of 1907 some agreements had been worked out; these included the concession from China allowing the Japanese to reconstruct the "light railway," made for military purposes, that ran from Antung (Dandong) on the Korean border to Mukden and also the formation of a joint Sino-Japanese forestry company to develop timber resources along the Yalu River. More important, however, was a "secret accord" that allowed China to build railways between Ch'ang ch'un and Kirin but also prohibited the construction of any parallel or branch railway to compete with Japanese interests in the South Manchuria Railway. This last point soon resulted in renewed disagreements between China and Japan as railway development moved ahead in Manchuria.

CHINESE POLICIES IN MANCHURIA

For the traditional Chinese, Manchuria has always been regarded as not quite part of China. Although Manchuria was the ancestral land of the ruling Qing dynasty, the Chinese government in the late nineteenth and early twentieth century was vigorously engaged in new policies for developing and integrating the region into the Chinese mainstream. A key element in China's Manchurian strategy was the railway.

The railways were seen as a way to exploit the natural wealth of the Manchurian heartlands as well as balance the various foreign pressures on China. In the nineteenth century, China's relations with the external powers were managed by a system of multilateral treaties to maintain an equilibrium between competing interests, the age-old Chinese diplomatic approach of "using barbarians to manage barbarians." By supporting an Open Door Policy, to use the favorite American term, China tried to facilitate trade under Western rules while obstructing territorial ambitions of the external powers, thus maximizing commercial gains while minimizing long-term political and military commitments.[39]

The basic Chinese strategy in Manchuria and the other northern border areas was aimed at curbing Russian and Japanese influence, both by promoting colonization by the majority Han Chinese and by co-opting local Manchu and Mongol ethnic groups. This policy of colonization was congruent with China's vision to "develop" Manchuria, especially to encourage transition from nomadic pasturing to more productive sedentary agriculture.[40] The railways in the early part of the twentieth century provided new life to this ongoing policy for the borderlands. Not only were Chinese immigrants from the south needed for railway construction, but migration of agricultural workers, itinerant fur trappers, and petty merchants from across the Pechili gulf added to the growing population of Han Chinese settlers, thereby sinicizing the traditional homeland of the Manchus.

As a result of the death of both the Empress Dowager (Tz'uhsi; pinyin Cixi) and the Kuang-hsü emperor in 1908, the political leadership in China was in disarray. The previously selected emperor ascended the throne as a child but with the government in the hands of his twenty-six-year-old father, Prince Ch'un, as regent. Prince Ch'un was widely regarded as not up to the job, and he immediately filled his government with trusted family, friends, and long-time subordinates. Thus, the leadership in Manchuria turned over, too. In 1909 Hsi Liang (Xiliang), a rather austere but highly respected Qing official of Mongol ancestry, was appointed governor-general (viceroy) in Manchuria. Although Hsi was a Mandarin in the classical tradition, he was able to form cordial relationships with foreigners and was viewed in context as one of the more progressive of the Qing officials.[41] Hsi Liang immediately realized that his main task was to manage Russian and, especially, Japanese behavior in Manchuria. The Japanese had imposed their own interpretation of the Treaty of Portsmouth and the Sino-Japanese Agreement of 1905 and were moving ahead with their policies of covert colonization in Manchuria. Various disputes lingered on, unresolved, and this provided opportunities for growth of Japanese influence.

A key dispute between China and Japan involved the railway project to upgrade the line between the Korean border at An-tung to Mukden (the capital of Feng t'ian [Liaoning] province), the so-called An-feng line. On one hand the proposed upgrade of the line to a standard gauge would have obvious commercial benefits to Manchuria, but it also provided an additional route for sending Japanese troops into Manchuria from Korea, which by then was under almost total Japanese domination. A literal reading of the treaty, advocated by Hsi, allowed only the "improvement" of the line, not a "reconstruction" as desired by the Japanese. Hsi also sought an agreement from the Japanese to remove all Japanese troops and police from along the An-feng line. In short, Hsi was aiming at a Japanese demilitarization of Manchuria. Unfortunately, Hsi did not receive strong support from his superiors in the Wai wu pu (Foreign Affairs Ministry) in Peking, and he was forced to accept most of the Japanese interpretations of the 1905 agreement in his negotiations with the Japanese consul general in Mukden.

Unable to block Japanese influence by such diplomatic means, he turned his efforts to strengthening the Chinese side of things. Hsi Liang immediately developed a plan for a major banking initiative that was to have internal Chinese railway development as its major focus. Because Manchuria was too poor to generate the needed funds, Hsi Liang sought foreign loans for this project. This proposal was eventually approved in Peking and became an instrument, again, for balancing foreign powers against one another. In his colorful words: "If we do not build another railway apart from the railways of the two countries [Russia and Japan], we will not be able to save ourselves from disaster. It is as with man's body—when the vessels are cut, the members and the trunk exist in vain and there is no way to make them live."[42]

Hsi Liang's drive for foreign investment was, in his view, essential for the survival of China's economy as a great power. Not only did he envision railway expansion as a key element of infrastructure, he also advocated for currency reform.[43] The tortuous and intricate negotiations, both transparent and murky, that these efforts involved are interesting but not central to this story. In the end, several contingencies conspired to frustrate these heroic efforts: the fall of the Qing government; the Chinese misreading of the American bankers; and the fact that both Hsi Liang and his American counterpart in these negotiations, the interesting "Old China Hand" Willard Straight, got ahead of their constituencies in terms of policies and commitments.[44]

Thus, long past 1907, the date for implementation of the terms of the Treaty of Portsmouth, the major transportation routes in the three eastern provinces of China remained under the control of three separate governments: Japan, Russia, and China. The United States had a major stake in the future of Manchuria through its Open Door Policy, an ideal not fully realized. And China was in control of its own territory in name only. It was in this troubled region in those troubled times that the plague in its most virulent form would soon erupt with a vengeance not seen for centuries.

CHAPTER THREE

The Plague

With occasional outbreaks of plague as the norm, it is not surprising that the start of the 1910–1911 epidemic in Manchouli went
unnoticed at the beginning. The only descriptions we have are
based on the Russian railway authorities in Manchouli, but they
provide a picture of an initial routine problem that quickly esca-
lated out of control. The sole means for control of plague at the
time was isolation and various levels of quarantine of large populations of suspected cases. At the beginning of the epidemic, the Russian presence in Manchouli consisted of nine physicians, twenty-
six assistants, and seventy-six nurses, and other health workers.[1]
Sporadic cases of the bubonic form of plague were observed from
time to time in this region, but for the entire year before the great
epidemic, there were no cases observed in the railway zone, in
Mongolia, or in the Transbaikal district of Siberia. As early as September 1910, however, there were rumors of a blood-spitting disease among the marmot hunters in the area around Manchouli,
and on Tuesday, 25 October, Russian doctors in Manchouli examined two Chinese with "inflammation of the lungs"; during that
night, one patient died.[2] An autopsy and bacteriological analysis

was done in Manchouli, and a diagnosis of pneumonic plague was made. On Wednesday, 26 October, nine more Chinese were found dead, apparently from the same disease.[3] On 27 October the Russian authorities in Manchouli responded by notifying the international diplomatic representatives along the railway line as well as instituting surveillance procedures: a special sanitary executive committee was appointed in Manchouli and an observation station was set up to monitor suspected contacts with plague cases. The two available diagnostic criteria were elevated temperature, that is, fever, and hemoptysis (coughing of blood). Initially, these contacts were placed in an isolation ward in the Chinese Eastern Railway hospital, but by 1 November, with 270 people in quarantine, it became necessary to convert several railway cars into temporary isolation housing.[4] These freight cars were kept at a dead-end railway track and housed 25 people each. If there were no deaths in five days, the detainees were released, but if someone became ill, the patient was transferred to the hospital, the remaining inmates transferred to another freight car for an additional observation period, and the original car was disinfected.

The surveys of the Russian sector were undertaken twice daily by six of the Russian doctors while the Chinese prefect made a list of the Chinese inhabitants and appointed Chinese agents to search out plague cases in the Chinese sector and report them to the Russian medical committee. Because of overcrowding in the Chinese sector and because there were many unemployed or itinerant Chinese, this task was doubly difficult. Between 25 November and 10 December, more than fourteen hundred unemployed Chinese were sent to an even more remote location, the town of Tsitsihar (Qiqihar) about sixteen miles away, while the richer Chinese were merely placed in isolation in Manchouli. Still, the cooperation of the Chinese citizens especially was half-hearted at best. Not understanding the reason for isolation and quarantine, they resisted such measures. Sick people as well as corpses were abandoned on the street, making it nearly impossible to trace contacts. Further, many Chinese refused the unfamiliar oral thermometer used to detect fever. Sometimes, as a test, the doctors would ask people to quickly evacuate one of the railway cars used for isolation, and anyone moving slowly at such a welcome opportunity was investigated for illness. Such was the primitive screening necessitated by the burgeoning epidemic. Little by little, with these measures in place, the daily death counts gradually declined. By 22 December 1910 the last of the quarantined were released in Manchouli.[5] An estimated 483 deaths occurred in and around Manchouli as documented by the Russian railway physicians, but it was assumed that there were more fatalities beyond the railway concessions never reported.[6]

From the beginning, the epidemic was seen as taking the pneumonic form rather than the more usual bubonic form. Later in the epidemic, some confusion arose over this issue. Even though at this early time when it was believed to be pneumonic plague, measures aimed at rats (carriers of the flea vector of the bubonic form) were routinely instituted.[7] Based on their knowledge of endemic plague in the Amur River region, the local Russian physicians immediately suspected the tarbagan as the source of this outbreak. The American consul in Harbin, Roger Greene, noted at the outset the recent changes in the intensity of marmot hunting driven by recent demand for marmot fur in Europe: "Large quantities of the skins have been shipped to Europe in the last few years, and the prices offered for them have risen so fast that great numbers of Chinese have been attracted to the business of catching the animals."[8]

The story of the epidemic from this point on is really a story of three cities, three governments, and three systems. As the epidemic spread along the new railroads of Manchuria, it encountered first the Russian city of Harbin, next the Chinese city of Mukden, and finally the Japanese city of Dairen (formerly known by its Chinese name, Dalian). It is not simply symbolic that the Chinese city was sandwiched between the Russian and the Japanese presence in Manchuria. In a very real sense, this arrangement captured the essence of the geopolitical game of the time.

The Russian railway officials in Manchouli realized immediately the potential for spread of the plague by infected passengers and tried to isolate the first two cars of a mail train from Hailar (a town nearer to Manchouli) to Harbin, but somehow "the message went astray."[9] Although the next train into Harbin was, indeed, intercepted by the police, and the cars put on a siding so that more than seventy Chinese could be examined (no disease was detected), the microbe may have already made its way to Harbin.

PLAGUE REACHES HARBIN

Harbin, as the "Russian capital of the Far East," was better equipped than the rude frontier station of Manchouli to deal with catastrophe, medical or otherwise. On the other hand, it had a larger, diverse population of Chinese, Japanese, and Russians, with a sprinkling of Germans, Austrians, Greeks, and Turks.[10] Divided into two main sections, "New Harbin," or the Russian and international quarter, and Fuchiatien, the Chinese quarter, the city was still trying to resolve the competing and overlapping roles of the Russian railway administration and the Chinese civil government administration in the running of the city. The delicate diplomatic choreography in this contested region complicated the responses to stresses that demanded unity of action and policy. Most of Harbin was built up within the "Railway Concession," that is, the lands granted by the Chinese government to the Chinese Eastern Railway Company, which was under Russian administration. The rest of the city, including Fuchiatien, was under the administration of the layered bureaucracy of the Qing government. Locally, there was a Chinese official, the Tao-tai, functionally equivalent to a mayor, in the Western sense, but acting as the representative of the provincial governor rather than as an elected local official.[11] This system provided a direct link from local government to the Imperial government in Peking through the provincial governor, and, in the special case of Manchuria, by way of the viceroy, who presided over the three Manchurian provinces in the name of the court in Peking. On the other hand, the Russian administration was a mix of civil railway officials and Russian military officers. Usually, the system functioned at a basic level because of the bilateral recognition that the military power of the Russian presence was balanced by the legitimate moral authority of the Chinese government.

The American diplomatic presence in Harbin was represented by Roger S. Greene II (1881–1947), who would later become the director of the China Medical Board of the Rockefeller Foundation.[12] Greene's regular biweekly consular reports from Harbin to the United States secretary of state chronicle the evolving state of affairs in Harbin. On 12 November 1910 he reported that the first death from plague in Harbin had occurred on 9 November. By the next day the Russian railway authorities informed Greene that eighty-five people in Harbin were "under observation." He also reported that "the laborers' barrack, where the first Harbin case was discovered, was burned down, first being surrounded with wire netting by means of which all the rats escaping from the house were stopped."[13] In this first American notification about the plague in Harbin, Greene was already alerting Washington to the political implications of the plague in Manchuria. He noted that the German consul had issued an order requiring all German subjects and protégés (mostly Turkish subjects whose government was being represented by Germany) at Manchouli to comply with the sanitary committee there. The principle of extraterritoriality seemed to require each country to independently approve and ratify, for its own citizens, the policies and actions taken by the Chinese municipal authorities trying to control the plague.

One month into the epidemic, on 25 November, the day after the American Thanksgiving holiday, Greene wrote in the crisp formality of diplomatic dispatches, "I have the honor to report that the epidemic continues and appears to be spreading."[14] He especially noted:

> In Fuchiatien the situation is becoming serious. Although the services of a Russian physician [Dr. Roger Budberg-Boenninghausen] have been secured to supervise the work of combating the disease, the isolation of patients seems to be very imperfectly arranged for and it would be a Herculean task to put the town in a proper sanitary condition. The Tao-t'ai of Harbin has just informed me that up to the 23rd instant there had been twelve deaths in Fuchiatien and he had just received information of four more deaths on the 24th. He said a sanitary committee made up of representatives from all classes of residents of the town had been formed and compulsory cleaning had been enforced, while two Russian medical men and ten old-school Chinese doctors had been retained to look after the patients.[15]

Greene continued his report alerting the secretary of state, Philander C. Knox, that the Russians were considering cutting off all communication between Fuchiatien and Harbin. He noted that the Harbin daily newspaper (said to be independent of the Russian government), *Novaya Zhizn*, "urges the Russian government to introduce into Manchuria a sufficient number of troops to enforce the adoption of satisfactory sanitary measures" (fig. 6).[16]

By mid-December, the Russian authorities, who had a reputation for being rather diplomatic with the Chinese, seemed to be out of patience: the Russian civil governor, General Affanasiev, published in the Russian press a list of antiplague measures that included a military cordon around Fuchiatien, the Chinese section of Harbin, as well as the threat of death to violators of the cordon.[17] Although this list was later labeled "only a proposal" by Affanasiev, who noted that it did not have a timetable for implementation, it met with strong disapproval from both the Chinese and the non-Russian foreign community in Harbin. The Chinese Tao-tai (Yu Si-hsing) objected that he had not even been consulted and that such a cordon certainly violated Chinese sovereign rights. The British and American consuls were concerned that the "shoot on sight" provisions were unnecessarily endangering the foreign nationals under their protection: The British consul, H. E. Sly, "felt compelled, without approving of the remainder of the Notification, to take objection to the adoption of a measure which might expose the lives of British Subjects to danger. The exact meaning of the somewhat indefinite phraseology of the Notification was, of course, that any person acting in the manner stated would be liable to be shot or bayonetted."[18]

The main task confronting both the Russian and Chinese authorities was enforcement of quarantines and population movements. Their strategy was to segregate the infected from the healthy, the potential carriers from the unexposed population. With the only reliable indication of plague infection being the symptoms and signs of impending death, the medical authorities resorted to the simplest measures possible under the pressure of a massive epidemic: they quarantined groups of potentially exposed

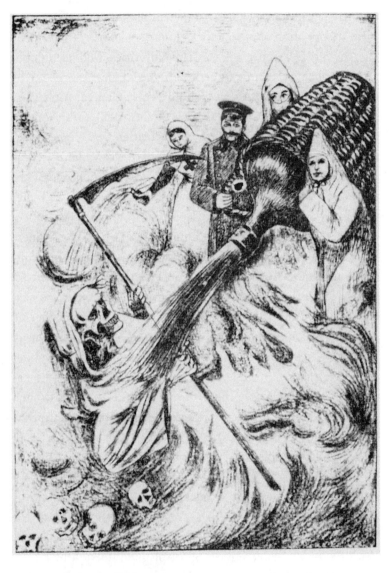

Figure 6. "We Have Won." Russian newspaper illustration.
(From *Novaya Zhizn*, Harbin, 1911)

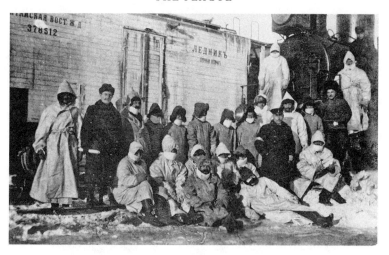

Figure 7. Plague workers in Harbin.
(From Thomas H. Hahn Docu-Images)

individuals for several days; if no cases developed in that group, all the individuals were deemed to be uninfected and could be safely released. The need for a large number of quarantine places was met by using railway cars to accommodate several dozen people for five to ten days at a time (fig. 7). Of course, if a case of plague occurred in one of the railway cars, it meant nearly certain death for all those in that car, because confinement in close quarters under the inhospitable conditions that prevailed in these make-shift accommodations was sure to maximize the spread of the disease. After release from quarantine for the lucky ones, each person was "tagged" with a wire wristband fastened with a lead seal, indicating that he or she had been quarantined, examined, and certified plague-free and hence was allowed to resume normal activities (fig. 8).

The Russian railway administration imported additional medical personnel from near and far. Some, including medical

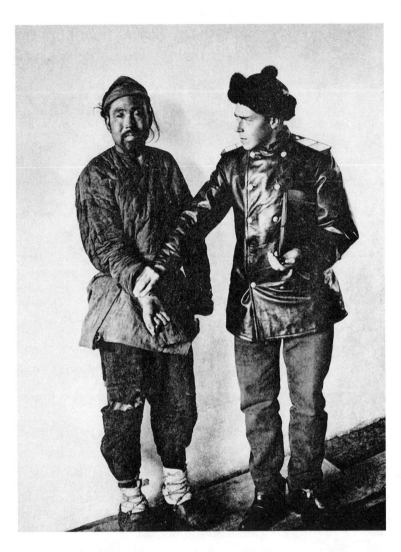

Figure 8. Chinese worker after a five-day detention and observation, with a wire and lead seal on his wrist showing that he has been checked for plague. He is accompanied by a Russian official. (From *Chuma v Manchjurii v. 1910–11 g.g.*; courtesy of the New York Academy of Medicine Library)

students, came from the famous medical college at the Imperial University of Tomsk in Siberia. Others, such as the leading Russian authority on plague, D. K. Zabolotny, were summoned from as far away as St. Petersburg.[19]

A main concern of the Russian authorities was the possibility of plague spreading eastward to the Russian seaport of Vladivostok. Probably for this reason, they focused their antiplague measures on containment at the Manchurian border and at their railway center at Harbin. In early February 1911, after the plague began to abate in Harbin and Manchouli, but when it was still raging elsewhere in Manchuria, the Russians convened a plague conference in the city of Irkutsk in Transbaikalia. The goals of this conference seemed twofold: to share information among Russian medical personnel who had been working in the plague regions along the Chinese Eastern Railway and to recommend procedures to limit the spread of the plague both eastward and westward along the railway route.

The Irkutsk conference ran from 7 to 14 February 1911 and was an archetype of cross-purposes. After hearing reports from physicians from the "front-lines" of the epidemic, as it were, the realities of commerce, financial resources, and government politics took over. While most of the medical personnel favored closing the border to train travel between Russian and Chinese territory as one of the most effective methods of containing the plague, others argued that this would hinder Russian economic interests as well as Russian "progress" in establishing its hegemony in Manchuria. Some proposed allowing border crossings by people who had undergone medical examination, but this entailed unacceptable medical expenses. At one point a vote was taken on the proposal to close the border: it failed, thirty-five to sixty. The financial support for the antiplague campaign was also debated:

up to this point most of the finances for fighting the plague came from city resources and some railway finances that were provided to the Antiplague Commission. The conference was able to agree that the Russian state coffers should be tapped for further funds to support the antiplague work.

The Russian conference at Irkutsk ended on 14 February with everyone dissatisfied. Since the majority of the participants were from Irkutsk, an apparently safe distance from the infected region, they lost interest in the urgency of the problem. The conflicting interests of the government authorities and the medical workers in the field were not resolved. Although a total of sixty-three articles were adopted by the conference, their scope and impact were weak and probably too little, too late. These provided for limiting travel into Russia (westward along the railway) which was to be allowed only at selected observation points, a five-day quarantine for most such travelers, disinfection of tarbagan skins from unknown regions, and retention of existing rules relating to export of leather, furs, animals, and food from plague regions. Interestingly, the conference also recommended an anti-rat campaign in the infected regions. Additional articles dealt with such matters as removal of convicts from infected regions, mandatory separation of passengers and cargo on ships, and the recommendation that immigrants be transported in railway passenger cars rather than in heated freight cars "as usual."[20]

While the Russian antiplague effort in Harbin was led for the most part by the doctors of the Chinese Eastern Railway, Chinese authorities in Harbin were active, too. The regional official in charge of Harbin in November at the beginning of the outbreak was the Tao-tai Yu Si-hsing, who served under the viceroy based in Mukden. While Consul Greene did not hold Tao-tai Yu in very high regard, Yu at least seemed to appreciate the gravity of the situation in Fuchiatien and engaged a Russian physician fluent in Chinese and familiar with local customs.[21] The viceroy in Mukden also took notice of the growing catastrophe and in early December 1910 sent one Chinese and one Japanese physician, both trained in Western medicine, to take charge of the medical work in Fuchiatien. The Japanese physician was reluctant to begin work until he was provided with the necessary equipment and authority, but once these were arranged, he apparently began work in the Chinese part of the town.[22] With the Russian threat of a military cordon around Fuchiatien, the Chinese authorities accepted Russian "supervision" of the Chinese sanitary measures in Fuchiatien by having one CER physician and one member of the Harbin City Council join the Fuchiatien sanitary commission.[23] The Chinese were particularly sensitive to both Russian and Japanese military threats of any kind: as Greene succinctly reported, "The situation here is complicated by the fact that the Chinese fear that if they invite Russian sanitary assistance, it will result in Russian police control in Fuchiatien."[24]

The Chinese physician sent by the viceroy in Mukden was Dr. Wu Lien-Teh (1879–1960), an ethnic Chinese born in Penang in the Federated Malay States.[25] His well-to-do family sent him to be educated at Cambridge University in England, after which he studied medicine at Saint Mary's Hospital in London. Following graduation he spent a year working with Ronald Ross at the Liverpool School of Tropical Medicine, then spent time at the Pasteur Institute in Paris and the Bacteriological Institute in Halle, Germany. At age twenty-four he completed his M.D. degree at Cambridge with a thesis on tetanus. Unable to find a research position back home in British Malaya, he ended up in private practice in Penang. Because he was an advocate of social reforms, such as elementary education for girls, removal of the queue, abolition of gambling, spirit licensing, and especially suppression of opium addiction, he was branded as dangerous and anti-British by the colonial government. His practice dwindled so that in 1907 he accepted an offer from China to be vice-director of the Imperial Medical College at Peiyang University in Tientsin (Tianjin), one of the schools recently established to educate Chinese students in Western medicine.[26]

In late December 1910, Wu and a senior medical student named Lin Chia-Swee arrived in Harbin. Lin was particularly valuable because Wu, as an "overseas Chinese," was not fluent in Chinese, especially the local dialects. Indeed, his Western ways, such as his preference for English and Western dress, seemed to rankle some of his Western colleagues in Harbin.[27]

On his third day in Harbin, Wu managed to do a limited post-mortem examination on a woman who had just died, and he was able to observe massive infection of her lung, heart, spleen, and liver caused by bacteria displaying the morphology and staining characteristics of Yersin's plague bacillus. He was thus firmly convinced of the pneumonic nature of the epidemic. While both Wu and most of his Russian colleagues in Harbin seemed to agree that the plague was not bubonic in form, both medical and diplomatic reports as well as certain sanitary practices, such as anti-rat campaigns, suggested lingering confusion on this important point.

Even with the arrival of Dr. Wu and his team of Western-trained physicians, the antiplague work in Fuchiatien still had its ups and downs. As the British consul Sly reported at the beginning of February 1911, "In Fu Chia Tien, the work of fighting the plague is proceeding more systematically and energetically and hopes are entertained that no inconsiderable improvement will soon be shown."[28] As one concrete example of this improvement, he noted Wu's having obtained permission for the cremation of corpses as a major step forward. Consul Greene, however, was not so sanguine:

> With two or three exceptions the inefficiency and neglect of the Chinese so-called foreign trained doctors and medical assistants is said to be appalling. Although provided with an ample number of assistants, the medical officers in charge of some of the newly-organized precincts, when called upon for their daily reports, have on some occasions been unable to show that they have done any real work in the line of inspection, discovery of cases and deaths, detention of contacts, etc. At the same time over 100 deaths were occurring in the city every day. Many of these men, who are supposed to report at 9:30 A.M. and to continue work till 4 or 5 o'clock in the afternoon, do not actually get to work till about noon, and then they frequently leave at two or three. There is reason to believe also that waste and corruption in the handling of official funds has reached very serious proportions.[29]

Some foreign observers in Harbin were unimpressed by the Chinese attitude toward the plague: they noted the prevalent Chinese theory that the plague resulted from having to smoke inferior grades of opium because of the recent campaigns to suppress opium in the Chinese empire. This theory neatly explained the high affliction rates of poor Chinese who could afford only cheap opium on the black market, and the sparing of wealthy Chinese who could afford the high cost of good opium.[30] Paper money, both Chinese and Russian, was suspect as an agent of transmission of the plague, too. It was subject to stringent sterilization by superheated steam, while coins were treated with corrosive sublimate (mercuric chloride).[31]

By the end of January 1911, the Chinese effort at plague control in Fuchiatien involved 20 physicians plus 25 Chinese medical students from either the Peiyang Imperial Medical College in Tientsin or the Peking Union Medical College.[32] By mid-February, in

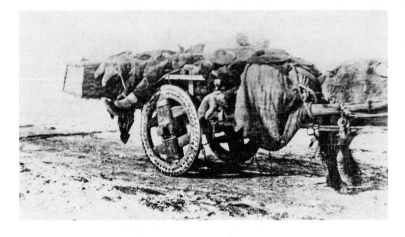

Figure 9. Overloaded wagon carrying the dead in Harbin, 1911.
(From Thomas H. Hahn Docu-Images)

Harbin, the epidemic was beginning to wane, whether because of the antiplague measures of the Russian and Chinese authorities or for other reasons. The deaths in Harbin fell from 35 per day in the last week of January to 27 per day in the first week of February and to 21 per day in the second week of February, with the corresponding figures from Fuchiatien being 147 per day, 119 per day, and 74 per day, prompting Consul Greene to report that "the situation seems to be really improving at Fuchiatien, for not only is the mortality diminishing, but better inspection and control is evidently being introduced" (figs. 9 and 10).[33]

PLAGUE IN MUKDEN

Although the plague seemed to be waning at the frontier and in Harbin, further south along the railroad from Harbin to Dairen, at Mukden, the plague was just starting to make itself known. Mukden, the ancestral home of the Manchus, was the most Chi-

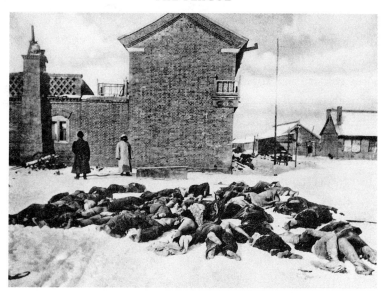

Figure 10. Corpses accumulated during a twenty-four-hour period outside a hospital in Fudzyadzyan, one verst (two-thirds of a mile) from Harbin. (From *Chuma v Manchjurii v. 1910–11 g.g.*; courtesy of the New York Academy of Medicine Library)

nese of the three principal towns along the route of the plague as it spread southward. Not only was it historically the most important to the Chinese rulers, it was the oldest town and the seat of the viceroy of the three northeastern provinces, His Excellency Hsi Liang. More important, it was the town where the Chinese could exercise the most authority in combating the plague. Mukden was at the juncture of the South Manchuria Railway under Japanese control and the Imperial Chinese Railway from Mukden to Peking, a rail line that was under undisputed Chinese control. Russia had lost control of the railway south of Ch'ang ch'un to the Japanese in the aftermath of the Russo-Japanese War, so there was only residual Russian influence in Mukden and Japan had yet to establish its presence there such as would come later upon its founding of the puppet Manchukuo state in 1932. The sanitary conditions in Mukden, its local government, and its medical institutions were more characteristic of an important Chinese town of that period, influenced by the practical Chinese politics of a region far from the center of such authority as the weakening Qing court could exert mixed with local and commercial interests, much of them Western in origin. While Harbin was a "company town" run by the railroad authorities with Imperial Russian backing, Mukden was a slowly modernizing old Chinese town with Western businessmen, medical missionaries, and Chinese bureaucrats sometimes working together and sometimes at odds to combat the growing epidemic that arrived with the new year.

On Monday, 2 January 1911, a sick traveler newly arrived from Harbin was found lying in the street in Mukden and was taken straight away to the government hospital. By the next day he was dead and the diagnosis was plague.[34] Dr. Wang Yu Shih, the Chinese medical authority in the city was short-handed because most of his staff had gone north to assist in the antiplague battle in Harbin. Surprisingly, he seemed to have made no advanced preparations in the likely case that the plague should spread to his city. Nonetheless, realizing at that point the need for aggressive measures, he started to organize his campaign against the plague in Mukden. Ten days later, on 12 January, he had assembled a small staff of medical students, police, and disinfection workers. The city was divided into seven districts, each with a plague office staffed by two medics, twelve police, ten disinfection workers, and several laborers to help with patient transportation.

House-to-house visitations started on 12 January, but because of the small size of the district staff, they concentrated on inspecting inns, lodging houses, and tea shops, places where transient Chinese were likely to congregate. The healthy areas of the town were visited every other day. Plague cases and their immediate contacts were immediately removed to a make-shift quarantine station in a small house in the western part of the city, and within a few days the Shah-Hsi Temple was being used instead. The rooms were small and badly lighted, but this structure was all that was immediately available as a temporary plague hospital.

On Saturday, 14 January, when the death rate in Mukden was still only 4 or 5 per day, the local authorities decided to close the Chinese Eastern Railway between Ch'ang ch'un to Mukden to prevent a continued influx of new cases from the north. That day the last train, loaded with migrant Chinese workers going home for the New Year, left for Shanhaikuan to the south. Two deaths occurred on the train and all 478 Chinese passengers were returned to Mukden the next day. Because the plague hospital and quarantine station could not accommodate such a large number of people, the passengers were housed in several inns near the railway station, with guards to prevent their leaving. These inns were crowded, poorly heated in the bitter Manchurian winter, and very dirty. Many of these workers died in the next few days. On the night of 23 January more than 100 of the surviving detainees broke out and escaped from the guards and could not be traced. Over the next week the death rate in Mukden rapidly increased, and Dr. Wang attributed this rise to the dissemination of the infection by those who evaded the quarantine. The next day, 24 January, the remaining inmates in quarantine were moved to the regular isolation station.

The medical supervision of the quarantine stations was risky yet undertaken by volunteer personnel from the local medical community as well as doctors and medical students who had traveled to Manchuria to assist in the epidemic. One particularly noteworthy early casualty was Dr. Arthur Jackson, a young English physician on the staff of the Mukden Medical College. Jackson had taken charge of the antiplague work in the railway area and on 24 January he became ill, was diagnosed as having pneumonic plague, and died the following day. His friends later memorialized him and his service in Mukden with a statue in that city as well as a laudatory biography.[35] The overall mortality rate for qualified doctors working in the antiplague effort in Manchuria was reported to be 5 percent, that of medical students was 3.5 percent, and for the entire population of antiplague workers, such as native practitioners, ambulance drivers, soldiers, and sanitary police, it was an astounding 10 percent.[36]

From the beginning, most of the deaths in Mukden occurred in the region known as the "seventh division," an area of inns for transients and roughly built hovels located between the center of the city and the railway station. The other divisions where most of the day laborers lived (the fifth and fourth) also experienced high death rates. The remaining four divisions were relatively unscathed by the epidemic. Local Chinese merchants, showing their civic responsibility as well as their concern for their businesses, decided to improve upon the official efforts to control the plague by raising money among themselves and opening an isolation hospital of their own. They engaged several traditional Chinese medical practitioners to manage this facility. The methods employed were based on the principles of Chinese medicine and did not include any direct attempts at antisepsis or other precautions against contagion. Within the first two weeks of its operation, this private plague hospital recorded 160 deaths, including 4 of the attending physicians. The death rates in Mukden for the week of 16–21 February ranged from 57 to 66 per day, with the majority occurring in this hospital. On 20 February the Mukden civil authorities managed to close this building.

With the railway lines into and out of Mukden closed, and the influx of migrant Chinese workers from the north markedly slowed, and with the closing of the merchants' hospital, the death rate began to subside. In the last week of February, only thirty-three people died of plague each day in Mukden, and for the first four weeks of March, the death rates fell even further, from daily averages of twenty-six to fourteen, then seven to two.

PLAGUE IN DAIREN

It is not surprising to find that the preparations and responses to the plague in the territories controlled by the South Manchuria Railway Company, the surrogate for Japan in Manchuria, were thorough, well-organized, and efficient, in marked contrast to the seeming haphazard Chinese responses in Mukden. The structures, both administrative and physical, put in place by the South Manchuria Railway reflected the political as well as the public health interests of its first director, Gotō Shinpei. No doubt because of its distance from the initial focus of the epidemic as well as the extensive measures taken by the Japanese in their Leased Territories in South Manchuria, the plague never reached Dairen, Japan's model city at the tip of the Liaotung peninsula. Instead, perhaps because of the blockade of the South Manchuria Railway route to Dairen and the ferries across the Bohai Sea, the populations carrying the plague were diverted onto the Chinese line from Mukden to Peking, which resulted in a spread southwestward along that line and away from Dairen and Port Arthur.

As soon as the plague was discovered in October 1910, the Japanese authorities in South Manchuria began planning for quarantine and hospital facilities in case they became necessary. At nine locations along the South Manchuria Railway, at main terminals, such buildings were erected or converted from abandoned Russian military barracks.[37] They were built to house between five hundred and five thousand detainees.

The Japanese established two lines of defense against the plague: an inspection program on trains and ships, and four sanitary cordons in layers around Dairen and Port Arthur.[38] Starting on 25 November 1910, the Japanese authorities began examining all travelers on trains embarking at South Manchuria Railway stations. Later, they instituted a seven-day observation period for all Chinese "of the lower classes (coolies, etc.)" who wished to travel on the railway. Many of the detained Chinese, however, did not understand the purpose of this quarantine and took to the roads on foot, walking south through the countryside and villages. The Japanese, in an attempt to stop this foot traffic, deployed both police and soldiers to control these Chinese travelers.

The firsthand report of one Captain von Kayser, master of the German vessel *Iltis*, gives a vivid picture of both the Japanese responses to the plague in Dairen as well as an assessment of its impact on the region and its people. This report was originally prepared for Governor Truppel, the official in the German concession of Kiaochow, and then translated and "officially leaked," confidentially, to J. C. McNally, the American consul in Tsingtau (Qingdao), for transmission to the United States secretary of state. Captain von Kayser's account, although somewhat abridged, is noteworthy for its objectivity, its detail, and its sense of immediacy:

> At 11 A.M. [24 February 1911], Captain Mersmann, Dr. Bengsch [physician aboard the *Iltis*] and I, accompanied by Mayor Yoshi-

mura [of Dairen] whom we met at the depot, the chief of police, Dr. Kitamura [a German-speaking physician from the South Manchuria Railway] and the Harbor captain went with the regular train to Ta fang shen (Daiboshin, Jap.) where the nearest of the three isolation camps is situated. At present there are three: In Changchun (for 3000), in Mukden (for 3000) and in Daiboshin (for 500 but will be extended to hold 3000). The camp of Daiboshin lies about 45 minutes with the railway from Dairen, close behind the Russian position of Nahshan [Nanshan] (Kinchou) near the railway. It consists of former Russian military barracks (brick) each for 25 men. . . .

The camp—surrounded by deeply sunk corrugated iron walls—is divided into two parts, which are also divided by corrugated fences. Part I is for the staff (among them 25 physicians) with a military guard, part II for sick and suspicious ones with a police guard. When leaving part II for part I one has to pass an electrically heated footscratcher, saturated with carbolic acid, and the hands must be washed in a mercury solution. The soldiers still wore masks, the attendants did not. The masks were formerly worn in Dalny [Dairen], until Dr. Kitasato declared them unnecessary and exaggerated. About 1000 Chinese had passed the camp so far, having to stop there for 7 days if coming from the North; one pest [plague] case had occurred. . . .

Remarkable was the extensive employment of Chinese as attendants, daily wage 35 sen—, the Japanese only acted as managers and oversee-ers.

At the outbreak of the pest in Dalny all non-infected Chinese of the infected quarters and blocks—regardless of position were brought in railway cars to this camp at Daiboshin. Here they remained 10 days (at other times only 7 days) as the Japanese at Mukden claim to have observed pest after the ninth day.

Right in front of Daiboshin the military cordon was drawn across the peninsula of Kinchou. During day time 6 guards stood in heated little block houses with windows (the territory was level and easily overlooked), at night there was lively patrolling. . . . The cordon is one English mile long. By the prompt use of the rifle a quick end was brought to attempts of Chinese to sneak through.

. . . Right after dinner [upon returning to Dairen] we drove to the pest hospital lying behind Osaka machi [a main road in Dairen]. During the drive one of the infected quarters was passed. The Chinese houses were cleared, nailed up; houses in which cases had occurred were burned down. The houses of the officials of the South Manchuria railway were protected against rats by corrugated iron sheets. . . .

The hospital at Daiboshin was divided into two parts. It contained amongst others a laboratory, presided by a scholar of Kitasato. Attendants: Chinese. At the hospital all rats are destroyed by fire. For the transportation of rats special boxes have been built.

The rat lottery has shown splendid success. Up to now 20,000 rats have been delivered. A specialist rat catcher has arrived from Japan.

. . . The hospital proper was a wooden structure, the houses of the attendants, as well as the morgue (with special corrugated iron wall,) were specially constructed brickhouses in barrack style.

From the hospital we drove to the near coast, outside of the closed harbor lying guarded compound.

The entire Chinese population of Dairen is at present housed in 4 such compounds. They live there with their wives and children and can follow their work freely, but are examined daily by four physicians stationed in the compound. (Puls [*sic*] and temperature). The compound near the harbor holds 5000 people. It is plain and had been built in three days, and is at present enlarged. (sketch) It consists of matsheds, for each 25 people one, (in reality there were probably 40–50 people in one.) inside to right and left were two kongs [*sic*], (Brick sleeping places), at the front side the cooking place. Each tent can be heated, and has a glass window at the rear side. Length about 15 meters, width on ground 4-1/2–5 meters, height 4 meters. The W.C. were as far as I could see, huts open toward the south with a wall in front.

The Chinese seem to feel well in the compound. They had moved without causing trouble, however, they have never been asked about it, but had to obey. The assistance of prominent Chinese was not required. The air in the huts was in spite of the outer cleanliness— simply mephitic.

Harbor and Ships.

The harbor territory is closed by a wire fence and the streets by wooden barriers. There is only one exit on the main harbor street. . . .

During the first pest days a disinfection room with carbolic vapors was being used which everybody had to pass. This measure was abolished after a few days. Seventeen thousand persons passed the gates everyday. There was no shortage of coolies in Dairen as the pest occurred before the Chinese new-year. . . .

All ships had to be disinfected and sulphured against rats. At present only sulphuring is required. Disinfection is said to have been done by means of a hot-steam apparatus placed upon a lighter. . . . No accurate news could be learned about this, nor could the lighter be inspected. . . .

Our reception can be considered accommodating and amiable. All measures of the Japanese bear the characteristic [thoroughness].[39]

As D. K. Kasai, who managed the preparedness in South Manchuria for the Japanese authorities, noted, "A cordon was drawn around the Kwantung territory from the east to the west coast."[40] All these preparations were in place at least a month before the plague was knocking at the door, so to speak, in Mukden. These coordinated, massive, and rather draconian measures, however, were no doubt effective: the combined death toll in Dairen and Port Arthur was only seventy-six.[41]

THE END OF THE EPIDEMIC

Mortality from the plague, wherever it occurred, began to diminish by the end of January 1911, perhaps because quarantine measures were working, perhaps because the cold weather limited population movements, perhaps because the Chinese New Year travels had subsided, or perhaps for other, more obscure reasons. Wu Lien-Teh dated the beginning of the end of the epidemic to a mass cremation of plague victims in Harbin on the last day of January 1911.

Dr Wu arranged with Dr. Chuan of the medical staff to engage 200 laborers and start work early the next morning [31 January] to col-

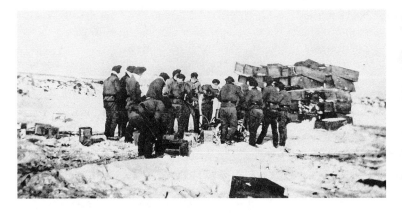

Figure 11. Stacked coffins waiting for cremation, with cans of kerosene nearby, Harbin 1911. (From Thomas H. Hahn Docu-Images)

lect the coffins and bodies and arrange them in tiers of one hundred. Mechanical pumps and hoses ordinarily used in firefighting were sent to the spot. Altogether twenty-two piles were raised. At two in the afternoon of January 31, some senior medical officers as well as a few selected civil and military officials were invited to watch the first mass cremation of infected bodies in history. Kerosene was pumped onto the piles, and when this method was found to be rather slow, the more intrepid labourers, who had become interested in the operation, asked to be allowed to climb to the top of the piles with tinfuls of kerosene and empty the contents from there. Permission was gladly given, and before the hour was out, every pile had received its share of paraffin. The order was given for fires to be lighted, beginning with the pile nearest the gathering and ending with the one farthest away. In a short order while the whole area was ablaze with burning coffins, all crackling and emitting black smoke. Photographs were taken [fig. 11] of the historic scene, and soon the tall piles could be seen slowly crumbling down to the ground which had become softened by the intense heat. Great was the elation and relief of everyone concerned at the climax of their efforts, and it was generally felt that the most effective day of their arduous campaign had been achieved by this great and historical operation.[42]

This bonfire was on the first day of the Chinese New Year for 1911, and Wu came up with yet another twist in his antiplague campaign. Part of the New Year tradition involved the explosion of firecrackers to celebrate the auspicious occasion. The Antiplague Bureau printed twenty-four thousand leaflets calling on the people of Harbin to celebrate the New Year by setting off the firecrackers *inside* their houses this year. One aim of the firecrackers was to disperse any evil spirits that might bring bad luck for the coming year, so Wu suggested that because the plague represented an extraordinary evil influence, it might take more than the usual diligence to rid their homes and belongings of the evil spirits. The scientific motive, however, was to exploit the sulfurous vapors from the firecrackers to disinfect the homes and reduce the presence of plague bacilli in the intimate surroundings of the population.[43]

For whatever reason, plague deaths continued to decline all during February 1911, without relapse, and the last case in Harbin was registered on 1 March 1911 with only scattered cases reported elsewhere until the end of March. Two Western visitors to Manchuria in May 1911 would poetically note: "Soldier, sailor, tinker, tailor, of half the races of the Occident and the Orient pass to and fro with gay laughter and chatter. Under the lovely purple evening sky of the East, diamond-powdered with scintillating stars, the concourse flows up and down the cobbled Kitaiskaia [the main street of Harbin, now Zhong Yang street]. It seems hard to believe that a very few short weeks ago this spot was the center of the most dreadful outbreak of pneumonic plague in the world's annals, the streets full of dead and dying, and the air foul with the drifting smoke of burning pits and a hundred smouldering houses, the only traffic that of the dead cart and plague van."[44]

In the final reckoning, the death toll stood somewhere between forty-five thousand and sixty thousand, the largest plague epidemic in modern times. Just what happened? Where did the epidemic start? Why was it so virulent? What were its consequences? Answers to these important questions would begin with the work of the International Plague Conference to be held in Mukden in April 1911.

THREE CITIES, THREE STYLES

The story of the plague and the responses to it as it moved south along the new rail system in Manchuria is a story in contrasts in styles: administrative styles, medical styles, and historical styles. Harbin was a brand-new town, a Russian town with strong European architecture and planning, strong central authority in the form of the quasi-military government imposed by the Russian railroad officials. Cordons were set up with shoot-to-kill orders. Quarantines were established with little effective resistance, and the layout of the town facilitated the segregation of the Asian population of Chinese and Korean workers from the European professionals, soldiers, and managers. Antiplague measures were undertaken quickly because the local Western physicians, mostly associated with the Russian railway company, at least had knowledge if not direct experience with small plague outbreaks in villages along the railroad in Transbaikalia.

However, Mukden and Ch'ang ch'un, the other main Chinese town on the railroad, were much less coordinated in their responses. They relied more on the local Chinese administration, a combination of officials and local gentry, to organize hospitals, approve quarantines, and otherwise implement the restrictive measures seen as unpopular with the population of Chinese workers. Mukden was old, an unplanned city, with traditions that were hard to disregard. Strong central authority was lacking. Western medical knowledge was missionary-based rather than company-financed as in Harbin. With a more diffuse geographic and administrative structure, one might have expected a weak response to the plague, but interestingly, the seemingly haphazard organization, which maintained sensitivity to local customs and a sense of autonomy, was able to maintain cooperation, implement reasonably effective quarantines, and deal with the pressures from both Russian and Japanese authorities. Without the nearly complete segregation of the populations seen in Harbin, the feeling in Mukden seemed less divisive and the surviving documents lack the ethnic edge of the Harbin accounts.

Dairen, as a new city, planned by the Russians, and later developed by the Japanese, was again not very "Chinese." The architecture and city layout were Western, and the administration was explicitly military, with some moderating influence of the public health doctor, Gotō Shinpei, who had been its early leader. Preparedness, organization, and efficiency were on display in Dairen, but, in fact, the plague never arrived in force to test the preparedness of this Japanese stronghold. Instead of following the main South Manchuria Railway line south to Dairen and Port Arthur, the plague penetrated southwest of Mukden via the Imperial Chinese line connecting Mukden to Peking, eventually to end with its surrender in the cold northern winter of 1911 near the tiny village of Suichun (Suizhong).

CHAPTER FOUR

The International Plague Conference
and Its Aftermath

ORIGINS OF THE CONFERENCE

As the plague gathered strength and continued its southward devastation along the railway routes of Manchuria, the de facto foreign governments in Harbin and Dairen perceived both the threat and an opportunity in terms of their national interests. The Japanese in the south saw the chance to solidify their already entrenched position in Manchuria by further extending their influence into the area of public health, quarantines, and other forms of population control. In the northern city of Harbin, the Russian authorities saw the plague as an opportunity to break out of their restrictions to the railway corridors and bring in additional Russian troops with the expressed purpose of enforcing quarantines and controlling travel and population movements. Predictably, the Chinese government, weak though it was, resisted these affronts to its sovereignty.

The United States seemed to be most concerned about the ambitions of Japan in Manchuria, and perhaps with good reason. In January 1911, at the height of the epidemic, the Japanese appeared to be preparing for both a troop buildup in Manchuria as well as an extension of their influence northward to Mukden. In the settlement of the South Manchuria Railway Company in Mukden, new barracks suddenly appeared that could accommodate three thousand troops. At twenty other locations along the South Manchuria Railway, additional such constructions were reported to be hastily erected. Although the stated purpose of these quarters was for quarantine of lower-class Chinese passengers on the South Manchuria Railway, the Chinese authorities saw these structures as potential housing for Japanese troops. At the same time, the Fifth Division of the Japanese Army, then in Hiroshima, was reported to be on its way to Manchuria to relieve the Eleventh Division. The Chinese, however, were concerned that a pretext might be found to retain the Eleventh Division in Manchuria, thereby doubling the Japanese military presence on Chinese soil. At the same time, Viscount Oshima, governor-general of the Leased Territory in the Liaotung peninsula, had quietly relocated his command headquarters from Dairen to Mukden under the guise of being chair of the Japanese Sanitary Commission, which was leading the antiplague work there.[1]

In early February, General Oshima met with Chinese viceroy Hsi Liang and suggested that China cooperate with Japan, allowing the Japanese to provide assistance along with Japanese experts as advisers. Although Viceroy Hsi was receptive to friendly cooperation from all sources, he made it clear that the administrative authority was entirely Chinese responsibility. Oshima urged Hsi to memorialize the Throne on this matter; the prompt answer from Peking was that Japanese cooperation in matters connected with Chinese administration could not be accepted. The Japanese, however, were not so easily dissuaded. The next day, the Japanese consul general called on Viceroy Hsi and insisted that the Chinese police cooperate with the Japanese police in visits to Chinese homes in search of plague cases. The viceroy responded firmly that the matter had been settled, and that all administrative power over Chinese territories outside of the South Manchuria Railway zone belonged exclusively to China. The Japanese consul general even went so far as to accuse the viceroy of acting in bad faith and again requested that the viceroy memorialize the Throne, which apparently he did.[2]

Viceroy Hsi confided to the American consul in Mukden that he was under heavy pressure from Japan to accept their proposal for increased administrative control in Manchuria, to which Fred D. Fisher, the American consul, responded with an alternative idea. He suggested that the powers cooperate with China to establish an International Sanitary Commission. Hsi Liang was receptive to this idea and since Fisher had lined up support from the British, French, and German consuls in Mukden, this suggestion was forwarded to the Wai wu pu (Foreign Affairs Department in Peking) for its consideration.[3]

At the same time the Russians had developed their own proposal for international intervention in Manchuria. On 19 January 1911, the Imperial Russian ambassador in Washington contacted Secretary of State Knox to propose that "the Chinese should intrust [sic] to foreign physicians the care of deciding upon such measures [to combat the plague], these physicians to be in the Chinese service." The Russian proposal went on: "It would be highly desirable to agree with the Chinese Government to have an international scientific expedition sent to Manchuria with object to study the centers of bubonic plague and to report on progress of the epidemic."[4] The next day Knox wired his support of this proposal to Peking, St. Petersburg, and the United States surgeon general, whom he charged with recruiting the experts to represent the United States.

China wasted no time in picking up on this suggestion, at least the part relating to a scientific expedition. On 22 January 1911, the Chinese sent telegrams to foreign governments, asking them "to send qualified Doctors to Harbin, thoroughly to investigate the plague and its causes. The traveling expenses and cost of maintenance of the Doctors so sent will be met by the Chinese Government."[5] The telegram to London that day was even more specific: the specialists are "to investigate the cause of the plague and to devise preventive remedies, and this way to advance Medical Science and at the same time safeguard human life." In contrast to the Chinese aim of "investigation," the Russian conception of this effort was basically administrative: an Imperial Prince residing in Peking would be appointed as high commissioner and would "act through the agency of special delegates in Manchuria placed under his direct orders."[6]

The Chinese, however, left nothing to the imagination. A few days after their first invitation to foreign doctors, they sent a follow-up telegram to the British ambassador in Peking: "The principle intention of inviting the several Governments to send doctors to Harbin is to investigate the conditions of the plague and to advance the Medical Art in dealing with it *but not to undertake executive work in carrying out preventive measures* [emphasis added]. You will again inform the British Government clearly of this point and ask them to send one specialist to come and take part in the investigation."[7]

For its part, Russia was also wary. It did not want the foreign experts treading on its turf either. On 27 January Count Benckendorff, the Russian ambassador in London, informed Sir Edward

Grey, the British foreign secretary, that whatever international body might be formed, it should not operate within the railway zones of the Russian-controlled Chinese Eastern Railway. This would be seen by Russia as an unacceptable assertion of Chinese authority in the railway zone should this happen.

The Russian Embassy in Washington sent a memo to the United States to reinforce its position: "It goes without saying that it shall be the duty of the physicians which either the Russian or any other friendly Power may send in aid to the Chinese Government to devote their work exclusively to Chinese territory outside the conceded zone of the Chinese Eastern railroad."[8]

For their part, the Chinese were concerned, too, about Russian intentions. On 31 January the secretary of the Chinese Legation in Washington, Yung Kawei, called the U.S. State Department to object to the Russian limitation that excluded the railway zones. "The Chinese Government believes that investigation under these circumstances is impossible because Harbin is a center of plague *and* the railroad."[9]

The United States did not let this situation pass without comment and on 9 February sent a note to both St. Petersburg and Peking: "This government's refraining from a discussion of the questions which may possibly be involved in your use of the phrase 'conceded zone of the Eastern Chinese Railroad' should in no wise be interpreted as implying any modification of the well defined views of the United States as to the situation apparently referred to."[10]

The Imperial Russian Government appeared careful to keep the United States government informed about its actions in China, perhaps trying to enlist the Americans on its side against Japanese aggressiveness. On 13 February Prince Nicholas A. Koudacheff, the Russian ambassador to China, sent Secretary of State Knox an outline of a Chinese-Russian agreement that included the following points: "1. Establish points of sanitary observation on the Chinese side of the Amur river; 2. Adopt, under Russian administration, in the Amur basin, coordinated measures against the epidemic along the rivers that traverse Chinese and Russian territories; 3. Sanitary examination in Chinese ports of laborers coming by sea to the Russian seacoast provinces; 4. Closure of opium and public houses on the right bank of the Amur facing Russian towns on the left bank."[11]

In this same communiqué, Russia assured the United States that it continued to respect Chinese sovereignty. The nature of the "points of sanitary observation," however, was open to varying interpretation: only six days later Knox received a telegram from the United States Legation in Peking indicating that Russian fear of the spread of plague into Siberia was leading to rumors that Russia was planning to establish military posts on the Chinese side of the Amur.[12]

PLANNING THE PLAGUE CONFERENCE

By the end of January 1911 the momentum for some sort of international consortium of "experts" to come together in China was building rapidly. The precise charge to this group and its aims were less clear. Russia was hoping for a body with administrative authority, while China resisted that role for such a commission. The United States, Great Britain, and France, the other active parties in this negotiation, seemed happy to see some opening to assist China on its own terms. The only question mark was Japan, which seemed silent on this proposal. Of course, Japan had the largest presence already on the ground, and its experts were already in China in the guise of South Manchuria Railway personnel and public health authorities in the Leased Territories.

Still, the proposal for an international scientific mission to Harbin provided China with a way to admit it was not up to the task of fully managing the epidemic alone, and that it would accept international help, albeit on its terms. The charge of "do nothingism" was thus deftly deflected without lost of sovereign face.

The international community acted quickly to identify "specialists" to send to China. Within two weeks, both the United States and Great Britain had recruited their representatives to the "Plague Commission in Manchuria," or the "Medical Congress for Investigation of Plague," as it was variably called. The U.S. surgeon general, Dr. Walter Wyman, reported to Knox that his service had an expert in Manila as well as one in San Francisco. The Navy proposed Dr. Edward R. Stitt of Canacao, Philippines, and Ambassador Calhoun in Peking suggested both Dr. Victor Heiser, director of the Philippine Health Service in Manila, and Dr. Charles W. Young, already in Ch'ang ch'un.

Word of this international commission spread rapidly. Dr. Martin R. Edwards of San Francisco wired the secretary of state to inquire about a "rumor" to the effect that three Pacific Coast states together with Harvard University were about to "help establish an institution to study plague and institute sanitary measures."[13] He presumably was ready to offer his services.

The State Department maintained close ties with the American Red Cross for informal diplomacy carried on under the banner of medical relief, and when Huntington Wilson, the assistant secretary of state, wrote to George W. Davis, chair of the Central Committee of the American Red Cross, he got a positive reply. After Davis consulted with the Rockefeller Institute for suggestions, Davis wrote to Surgeon General Wyman on 3 February to nominate Dr. Richard P. Strong and pledge three thousand dollars of Red Cross funds for Strong's use and support in China. This apparently clinched the deal, and on 9 February Strong became the official United States delegate to the, as yet to be clarified, China Plague investigation team.[14] Richard P. Strong was, at the time of his appointment, a member of the Bureau of Science, a United States government institution in Manila. He had been president of the Army Board for the Investigation of Tropical Diseases in the Philippine Islands, the forerunner to the Bureau of Science, and was a well-known expert in both cholera and plague.[15]

China had requested that Great Britain send Sir W. J. Simpson, their most famous plague expert who had worked on plague in both South Africa and Hong Kong. It was reported that Simpson asked for a stipend of ten thousand pounds, which the British government would not pay.[16] Instead, they settled on Dr. Reginald Farrar, of the Board of Health of London. It is not clear what his specific qualifications were for this assignment. He seemed to be concerned about the trip, and, in addition to asking for the usual support for travel and subsistence, he requested that the Chinese government insure his life for the sum of "say £1000." This latter stumbling block was left as a "matter for arrangement between his Dept and the Treasury."[17]

The British delegation was hampered by hurt feelings on the part of both the Lister Institute and the British Legation in Peking. Both appointed "unofficial delegates" to attend the conference as "observers." The Lister Institute sent Dr. G. F. Petrie, who at his own request to the Chinese government was appointed as an additional British delegate, and Dr. G. Douglas Gray, the British Legation physician in Peking who was also appointed as a

British delegate by the Chinese. According to Dr. Strong's post-conference report, these delegates frequently quarreled among themselves, presented different opinions, disagreed on which way to vote on matters, and finally disagreed on which one should sign the interim report. Dr. Petrie ended up signing it in the absence of Dr. Farrar. All in all, not a good show for the British.[18]

While the Japanese remained publicly aloof from these developing plans, the most famous Japanese microbiologist, Baron Kitasato Shibasaburo, head of the Institute for Study of Infectious Diseases in Tokyo, just happened to visit Manchuria on an inspection tour of the South Manchuria Railway on 17 February. His speech on plague, with special reference to the Manchurian epidemic, was published in English translation in Dairen. He emphasized the pneumonic nature of the present epidemic, noting that its control will be "an easy thing to accomplish from a scientific point of view" but went on to complain that the "best and simplest method [quarantine and population control] cannot be given full and free play, because of the environs of the South Manchuria Railway." These shortcomings were, he said, due to lack of cooperation of the Chinese authorities and population.[19] He also traveled to Mukden and on 20 February spoke informally to the diplomatic corps there at a meeting arranged by the Japanese consul, C. Keike.[20]

The Russian authorities had several options for its delegation: there were already experienced plague doctors in Harbin, some from the respected school of medicine in Irkutsk. Instead, Dr. D. K. Zabolotny, professor of bacteriology from the St. Petersburg Women's Medical Institute, who had experience with plague research in Odessa, was appointed to lead the Russian delegation. Strong characterized Zabolotny as a "pure scientist, a man who has apparently no political aspirations, and one who is not in sympathy with many of the political movements in his own country."[21] There were more than twelve members, both men and women, in the Russian delegation, of which only six were official delegates and four were deputy delegates.

Remarkably, either by design or accident, the powers seemed to acquiesce to the Chinese aim of restricting the international activities to scientific investigation rather than administrative maneuvering.

There are two particularly interesting aspects of events leading up to the arrival of the international experts in China. One is the confusion (or *apparent* confusion) surrounding the arrival of the American, Dr. Strong; the other is the posturing of the Japanese government with respect to the scientific respectability of the Chinese hosts.

When Strong was appointed as the U.S. representative, he was working in Manila in the Bureau of Science. On 12 February he received final instructions from Washington. He reported that he was "wanted in Manchuria immediately" and that it was impossible for him to wait until 15 March. On 14 February, the same day that Strong left Manila on his way to Peking, the Chinese government sent telegrams to the powers informing them that the "Plague Investigation Congress" would take place in Mukden, beginning on 3 April 1911 and was expected to last between two and five weeks.[22]

Strong was accompanied by his assistant from Manila, Dr. Oscar Teague. They had hastily assembled what laboratory equipment they could take from Manila and sailed for Shanghai. There, they bought all the guinea pigs that were available from the Municipal Laboratory under the direction of Dr. Arthur Stanley and traveled on to Peking. Finding, only upon arrival in Shanghai, that they were more than a month early for the congress in Mukden, Strong and Teague, with the concurrence of the U. S. ambassador, decided that they should go on to Mukden and begin their study of the plague well in advance of the scheduled congress. From the documents available, it appears that both the Chinese government and the U.S. authorities were quite aware that the congress would be held in April, but somehow Strong did not get this information and was under the impression that his services were needed in China as soon as possible. Without additional evidence, one can only speculate about the motives, if any, of the United States (or the Chinese, for that matter) wanting Strong in China long before the start of the congress. As Strong later reported, however, "This course subsequently proved to have been advisable." He explained that "upon our arrival in Shanghai and our receipt there of the telegram stating that the conference would not be held until April 3, and advising us to remain near Peking until the opening of the conference, it did not become clear to us why our services were required immediately in Manchuria, but it developed later that it was important for China that some other country, besides Russia and Japan, had sent representatives a sufficient time in advance of the meetings of the conference, and that these representatives had made original investigations and secured some favorable results."[23]

Later, he went on: "It seemed clear that the Japanese hoped that no other representatives would present work of any importance at the conference, and Japan sent three of her strongest scientific representatives, Professors Kitasato, Fujinami and Shibayama, as well as the staff surgeon general of her army and several other doctors to take part in this work."[24]

It thus appeared that Strong's "premature" arrival in China was arranged to allow China to balance the anticipated Japanese domination of the conference with the latest, most relevant research by the Americans done in collaboration with the Chinese in Manchuria.

The Japanese were worried that the conference might pass resolutions, in the name of the international community, that might limit their expansionist control of the South Manchuria Railway. They did not respond to the Chinese invitation, hoping that the absence of Kitasato, at the time believed by many to be the codiscoverer of the plague bacillus, would scuttle the meeting.[25] When it was clear that this tactic was failing, Kitasato accepted at the last minute but made several disparaging remarks about the ability and even the rights of the Chinese to contribute to the conference: "The Chinese authorities have no right to lay propositions before the Conference or to claim a voice in the Conference. Any attempt at either, if made by them would be highly improper and unpardonable and would be positively resisted by myself for one."[26] At the beginning of the conference on 3 April, the U.S. ambassador to Peking, William Calhoun, sent a coded telegram to the secretary of state summarizing the situation in Manchuria as "strained and delicate."

> The Japanese have all along been pressuring the Chinese to allow them to have charge of the sanitary work. The Chinese have been equally insistent in their opposition. The latter have worked very hard to control it [the epidemic] themselves and it is the consensus of opinion that all things considered they have done very well. The Japanese are apparently suspicious of or hostile to the medical conference now assembling. The Chinese were very much disturbed because for a long time they heard nothing from the Japanese Government in response to the invitation extended. The morning's advices are that while the Japanese delegate has arrived in Mukden he refuses to go to the quarters provided for the members but remains at a hotel by himself. Whether or not he will participate in the work of the conference remains to be seen.[27]

While the powers were lining up their delegations of experts, the Chinese government was making careful preparations for the conference in Mukden. Although Viceroy Hsi Liang was the official host for the Chinese government, the local arrangements for the meeting were put in charge of an imperial commissioner, Sze Sao-ke.[28] Sze, better known by the Western form of his name, Sao-Ke Alfred Sze, was a fortunate choice, both for his intrinsic talents as well as his experience in dealing with Westerners.[29] Sze had studied languages as a boy in China, was a student interpreter for the Chinese Legation in Washington, D.C., and had graduated from high school in the United States as well as from Cornell University (B.A., 1901, M.A., 1902). From 1908 until 1910 he had been the Tao-tai (circuit intendant) and customs superintendent in Harbin; not only was he well versed in Western culture, but he was intimately familiar with the Manchurian political landscape.

Strong and Teague arrived in Mukden on the evening of 27 February in the midst of a severe snowstorm. After several days of perfunctory meetings with the local U.S. consul, Fisher, and with Viceroy Hsi Liang, they set to work in three small rooms (formerly sleeping rooms for local workers) at the plague hospital in Mukden. With the implicit approval of the viceroy, they began to perform autopsies on the patients who had died of plague. Meanwhile, they sent to Berlin for an "Emergency Plague Laboratory" designed by the Koch Institute in Germany. This "kit" was shipped by express and was a self-contained trove of laboratory apparatus and supplies sufficient to carry out field investigations on infectious diseases.[30] The goal of their work was "the study of the way the disease was conveyed, its pathological anatomy, and its treatment." Strong further reported that "the study of the first two of these problems was pursued up to the time of the opening of the conference, and satisfactory results were obtained."[31]

Autopsies were obtained with difficulty and there was much local resistance to them. Finally, it was agreed that autopsies would be performed only on bodies that were unclaimed and unidentified. All in all, only twenty-five autopsies were done, but this proved sufficient to provide for the pathological-anatomical study of the disease. Indeed, these were apparently the first autopsies performed in Manchuria, and far more than any other conference participant had performed on pneumonic plague cases. By the opening of the plague conference, the Americans and their Chinese collaborators were in possession of substantial new and highly relevant information, enough, it turned out, to counterbalance the Japanese authority of Kitasato, Fujinami, and Shibayama.

THE CONFERENCE OPENS

The conference, by this time known officially as the International Plague Conference at Mukden, opened with a flourish on Monday, 3 April 1911. The Chinese government had lavishly spruced up an old palace called Shao Ho Yien (Little River Park) to provide living quarters, meeting rooms, and some laboratory space for the conference participants.[32] While most of the conferees stayed in this convenient, one-story modern hotel with electricity, running water, and most important, heat, the Japanese, for political reasons, set up camp in the Yamato, one of the flagship hotels of the South Manchuria Railway Company. The British delegates, likewise, decided to lodge with their own nationals in Mukden. The conference location was described as having a massive hall for the sessions of the conference with room for 150 people, a large dining room, and a main sitting room "with all the comforts of club life," including "the proverbial English afternoon tea [that] could be had at other hours than just four o'clock."[33]

Table 1. Key Participants at the International Plague
Conference Held at Mukden, April 1911 (From Strong, *Report
of the International Plague Conference*, vii–ix)

Dr. W. H. Graham Aspland, Professor, Peking Union Medical College

Dr. Dugald Christie, Director of the Mukden Hospital and Medical
Adviser to the Manchurian government

Dr. Ch'uan Shao Ching, Professor of Medicine, Therapeutics, and
Medical Jurisprudence, Imperial Medical College, Tientsin

Dr. Reginald Farrar, Local Government Board Inspector, London

Dr. Akira Fujinami, Professor of Pathological Anatomy, Imperial
University of Kyoto

Dr. Gino Galeotti, Professor of Experimental Pathology, Royal
University of Naples

Dr. G. Douglas Gray, Legation Physician, British Embassy, Peking

Dr. Paul Haffkine, Director of Russian Plague Hospital, Harbin

Professor Dr. Shibasaburo Kitasato, Director of the Imperial Institute
for Infectious Diseases, Tokyo

Dr. George Ford Petrie, Lister Institute of Preventive Medicine, Indian
Plague Research Commission, 1905–1907

Professor Dr. Gorosaku Shibayama, Chief of the Clinical Department,
Imperial Institute for Infectious Diseases, Tokyo

Dr. Arthur Stanley, Health Officer, Shanghai Municipal Council

Dr. Richard P. Strong, Professor of Tropical Medicine, Bureau of
Science, Manila

Dr. Wu Lien-Teh, Assistant Director, Imperial Army Medical College,
Tientsin

Professor Danilo Zabolotny, Professor of Bacteriology, St. Petersburg

Dr. Semion Ivanovich Zlatogoroff, Assistant Chief of Bacteriology,
St. Petersburg

Table 2. Countries Represented at the International Plague
Conference Held at Mukden, April 1911 (From Strong, *Report
of the International Plague Conference*, vii–ix)

China: 9 delegates and 8 deputies
      6 secretaries
      Alfred Sze, Imperial Commissioner of Wai Wu Pu
      Hsi Liang, Viceroy of Manchuria
Russia: 6 delegates, including two women and 4 deputies
Japan: 5 delegates
Great Britain: 3 delegates
Italy: 3 delegates
United States: 2 delegates
Austria-Hungary: 1 delegate
France: 1 delegate
Germany: 1 delegate
Mexico: 1 delegate
Netherlands: 1 delegate

At 10 A.M., Viceroy Hsi Liang opened the conference with
words of welcome. He conveyed greetings from His Imperial
Highness the Prince Regent, read in Chinese and interpreted by
Tsang Woo Huan, a translator from the Wai wu pu and one of
the conference secretaries. After what seemed to be conventional
sentiments from the regent advocating the delegates to "advance
the cause of humanity" and "throw much light upon the disease,"
the viceroy went on with his own lengthy remarks of a distinctly
modern flavor, in which he quoted the speech of King Edward VII
at the International Sanitary Conference in 1894: "If preventable,
why not prevented? . . . I trust and I believe, too, that modern
medicine, and especially sanitary science, will in [the] future re-

ceive more attention in this country than it has hitherto done, and that we shall be better prepared to deal with similar epidemics when they arise."[34]

Viceroy Hsi Liang was followed by Sao-Ke Alfred Sze, the imperial commissioner, who gave a welcome in English: he reviewed the "conditions which have produced the epidemic" and described the marmot link. He also laid out a list of twelve scientific questions (no doubt provided to him by Wu Lien-Teh) to be discussed during the conference. Sze also announced that Wu would serve as overall chair.

The final formal presentation was by Professor Zabolotny, who replied on behalf of the assembled foreign delegates. The meeting then adjourned until 2:30 P.M. the following day.

With Wu Lien-Teh as chair, a preliminary meeting restricted to official delegates was held at 2:30 P.M. on 3 April to adopt rules of procedure. English, German, and Chinese would be the official languages of the conference. A committee made up of Martini (Germany), Galeotti (Italy), and Teague (the United States) was elected (by ballot) to propose adjustments in the official program; another elected committee comprising Farrar (Great Britain), Zlatogoroff (Russia), and Shibayama (Japan) would meet "to arrange the daily work of the Conference." The minutes and reports of the conference were to be published in English.[35] In a deft diplomatic move, Wu proposed that Kitasato be elected "President of the Section on Bacteriology and Pathology." There were no other officially designated "sections," nor were there any other "presidents" elected. Kitasato's nomination was carried unanimously. One of the rules adopted, however, provided that whoever was occupying the chair of the conference should at that time be addressed as "Mr. President."

Perhaps because it would not be able to complete its work in time for the sessions to start the following day, or perhaps for other reasons, the French delegate, Broquet, with Kitasato's second, proposed that the program adjourn on Tuesday (the next day) immediately after the opening address by Wu Lien-Teh "as an act of homage to the doctors who lost their lives in Manchuria." This proposal was accepted unanimously.[36]

PLAGUE SCIENCE

The scientific program was a somewhat leisurely and informal mix of formal papers, hastily assembled "remarks," and long discussion sessions. Sometimes experimental results and demonstrations were presented for the delegates. The first scientific paper of the conference, significantly, was presented by Dr. Ch'uan Shao Ching, a Chinese physician of some rank who had been studying the epidemic on behalf of the Chinese government.[37] The paper was titled "Some Observations on the Origin of the Plague in Manchouli." From the outset he focused on the role of the tarbagans, the crowded camps for migrant trappers, and the generally unsanitary conditions in Manchouli, an approach later to be characterized as disease ecology. His detailed account of his on-the-spot investigations in Manchouli and his apparent identification of the index case in the epidemic provided the background as well as the foundation for much of the rest of the work of the conference. Other papers in this first session also focused not on the origins of this particular epidemic but on the historical role of plague in Manchuria. Dr. Gray, the British Legation physician, discussed plague in the northern regions of Manchuria, whereas Dr. D. K. Kasai, a Japanese physician from Dairen, discussed plague in the southern regions of Manchuria. Professor Zabolotny then summarized the Russian experiences with plague in the border regions along the Amur River.

The second section was chaired by Professor Kitasato, who introduced his session with the sweeping announcement that "we have now reached the most important part of the conference, namely the sections on bacteriology and pathology, and I think it would be best to enter upon these discussions at once."[38] Since this epidemic was recognized to have been "strictly" pneumonic in form, there was much interest in the possibility that a variant strain of the plague bacillus was at work here. Laboratory comparisons with other isolates as well as various animal virulence tests were reported. The roles of bacterial toxins and surface agglutinins were debated. These topics, the stuff of contemporary bacteriology, occupied the conference for several sessions. Kitasato must have been pleased that "his" sessions dominated the meeting.

Finally, the conference moved on to consider an array of clinical observations on the current epidemic. Modes of contagion (breath—no; coughing—yes; merchandise—no; household goods—yes) as well as diagnostic methods and criteria were discussed and observations debated. The existence of apparently healthy carriers was an important consideration; Dr. Dugald Christie presented one case report in which an apparently healthy person seemed to be responsible for at least three primary infections and indirectly for at least three more cases of the plague.[39] Addressing the theme of possible modes of treatment and prevention, trials of vaccine and serum therapy were described. The depressing conclusion of all these reports was that neither vaccines, such as killed bacterial vaccines as well as Haffkine's famous vaccine, nor Yersin's hyperimmune serum treatment had the least effect on the course of the disease once it was contracted. The role of vaccination in prophylaxis was unclear, but probably of minimal value as well.

As Dr. Strong pointed out in his presentation in the session devoted to "Morbid Anatomy," reports of autopsies done on pneumonic plague victims were hard to come by. Up to that point there had been only ten cases described in the world's medical literature. This epidemic provided an unprecedented chance to study the pathology of plague, and this opportunity was not lost on the physicians who traveled to China to study this epidemic. Strong reported on twenty-five autopsies done at Mukden, Fujinami reported on twenty-six cases from Ch'ang ch'un and Dairen (plus several donkeys), and Koulecha reported on twenty-eight cases (mostly on frozen and subsequently thawed bodies) from Harbin.[40] All three investigators described similar findings and reached the same general conclusions. There were the usual quibbles, but it appeared to all that the plague resulted in a lobar pneumonia, that it seemed to reach the lungs via the blood stream, and that the primary route of infection was via the throat or mucous membranes of the respiratory tract. Whether the tonsils and other lymphoid tissue were an important or only a secondary site of infection was a point of contention, however.

The final sessions of the conference were devoted to measures that were, or might be, used to combat the pneumonic plague. These sessions also included substantial statistical data on the plague's ravages in Manchuria: the number, locations, and timing of the cases, as well as the age distribution, nationalities, and social status of the victims. Several talks were of a general nature, reviewing attempts at control and therapy in prior epidemics, but there were extensive reports on the efforts of local officials as well as government agencies to contain and control the epidemic. The descriptions of emergency quarantine measures, hastily erected plague hospitals, and disinfection routines were presented for several of the hardest hit towns. In keeping with the powers' interest in Manchurian commerce, there were even reports on the economic impact of the plague on trade, agriculture, and railway traffic. Resolutions for both the use and further investigation of prophylactic inoculations were passed unanimously.

The scientific sessions were followed by a lengthy process of summing up, with the intent of formulating resolutions to be adopted by the conference as well as the preparation of an interim report on its findings. Four half-day sessions on 26 and 27 April were devoted to discussion of the contents and wording of the interim report. Finally, after a brief session on the morning of 28 April, at which Strong and Teague reported on their just completed study on the infection of tarbagans with the plague bacillus, the scientific sessions of conference adjourned.

The closing ceremony of the conference was held at 4 P.M. on Friday, 28 April 1911, with a reception and address by Viceroy Hsi Liang, presentation and acceptance of the Interim Report, a reply by Sao-Ke Alfred Sze, and a few concluding remarks by Wu Lien-Teh. The Interim Report was a short document (ten pages in Strong's conference report) with eleven "provisional conclusions" and forty-five "resolutions." Interestingly, none of the resolutions dealt with anything remotely political, as was initially feared by the Japanese. They instead dealt with suggestions for sanitary improvements and quarantine regulations. And finally, "In furtherance of the above purposes, every effort should be made to secure effective medical education in China."[41]

The final report of the conference was entrusted to an editorial committee consisting of Strong, Stanley, Martini, and Petrie. In addition to the material presented at the conference, the final publication has four chapters appended as "Part 3: Summary of

Knowledge Gained from the Study of the Epidemic." These summary chapters deal with epidemiology (Petrie), clinical and diagnostic features (Strong), bacteriology and pathology (Strong), and measures to combat the plague and its effects on trade (Stanley). Strong did the final editing of the report in Manila, and it appeared in the fall of 1911, printed there by the publisher of the *Philippine Journal of Science*—that is, the United States government.[42]

POSTCONFERENCE EVENTS

The elements of reform in the besieged Qing government were beginning to have some effect, and the success of the International Plague Conference perhaps did its part to strengthen their position. Sao-Ke Alfred Sze apparently used this opportunity to push for the establishment of a Chinese Scientific Research Institute in Peking. Shortly before the close of the conference, Sze approached Strong and his associate, Oscar Teague, to discuss the establishment in Peking of an organization modeled on the Bureau of Science in Manila. The Chinese were particularly interested in developing the biological side of the work, including bacteriological and hygienic work and the preparation of vaccines and sera, as well as chemical work aimed at both research and industrial ends.[43]

Sze noted that his discussions with Strong and Teague were to be considered confidential, because Sze feared that "if it became known that such an institute was to be established in Peking, . . . political influence would be brought to bear on his government, particularly by Great Britain, in which the appointment of candidates for positions in this laboratory would be urged. Some of these candidates might be undesirable, and this state of affairs he desired to avoid."[44]

Strong provided Sze with a rough estimate of the scope of the work, the staff required, and the amount of equipment that would be needed. Sze indicated that he could obtain an initial appropriation of 1 million taels ($650,000) for such an institute, which was within the range Strong had estimated for the undertaking.[45] With the approval and encouragement of their sponsor, the American Red Cross, Strong and Teague traveled to Peking after the conference for further discussions with Sze about such an institute. About a week later, on 8 May, Strong and Teague left for Manila with the understanding that Strong would be invited back to Peking "next Christmas" by the Chinese government and at that time be offered the scientific directorship of the institute. Strong was not inclined to move to Peking, but Sze was insistent, and so Strong did not entirely close the door on the possibility. Sze was open to other suggestions for the position. The Chinese, apparently, were particularly interested in staffing the new institute with American scientists: Strong noted that "it appeared . . . at the present time at least, a greater confidence was inspired in Americans than in other foreign advisors in at least certain branches of scientific work."[46] Strong, in his report to Secretary of State Knox, made clear his personal desire to remain in Manila but raised the question of "whether the State Department feels that it would be of particular advantage to American interests to have scientific control of this institute." Strong's Christmas trip, however, never materialized. The elements of reform and revolution swept away both the good and bad of the dying Qing regime in the fall of 1911. On 10 October the Wuchang uprising in Hubei province unleashed the Chinese Revolution that ended with the abdication of Emperor Puyi on 12 February 1912.

Sao-Ke Alfred Sze, ever the skillful diplomat, seemed to make the transition effortlessly. Before he could take up his new imperial appointment as minister plenipotentiary to the United States, Peru, and Spain, he was overtaken by the revolution led by Sun Yat-sen. In March 1912, however, Sze was appointed minister of communication in the new government, but he soon he resigned because of illness, later to become chief of protocol for President Yüan Shih K'ai. In 1914 he was appointed minister to the Court of St. James. His vision for a world-class scientific institute in Peking faded as China faced challenges even greater than the Manchurian plague.

JAPANESE AND CHINESE REACTIONS

The resolutions passed by the conference focused strongly on recommendations for improvements in China's public health organization, its medical education system, and its hospital and quarantine provisions. Both China and Japan took advantage of this momentum to develop new initiatives in Manchuria. Japan, through its quasi-official agent of colonialism, the South Manchuria Railway Company (SMR), established a new medical school in Mukden. China would use this occasion to implement the first steps toward a national public health system through the establishment of the North Manchurian Plague Prevention Service.

No sooner had the plague conference adjourned than the SMR submitted a request to the central Hygiene Office in Tokyo for permission to establish a "second level" medical school in Mukden. On 15 June 1911, the South Manchuria Medical College (Namman-igaku-do) was founded.[47] As a token to Chinese sovereignty, the new viceroy of Manchuria, Chao Erk-shun, was appointed honorary president; Kenji Kawanishi, the superintendent of the Railway Hospital in Dairen, was director of the new school. Like all Japanese medical schools, it was affiliated with one of the two key schools in Japan (Tokyo Imperial University or Kyoto Imperial University). In this case, the Mukden school was controlled and staffed by Kyoto Imperial University.[48]

The South Manchuria Medical College was the second medical college in Mukden; the other, Mukden Medical College, founded in January 1912, was run by Dr. Dugald Christie, a Scottish Presbyterian medical missionary. Although Christie had been training apprentices since 1892, he managed to build a teaching building adjacent to his hospital in Mukden in 1911 and started his five-year medical teaching program a year later.[49] While Christie's school, as well as the South Manchuria Medical College, was supported by foreigners with their multiple aims, they both admitted Chinese students (the Japanese school gave some preference to Japanese applicants, however).

The Chinese, too, saw opportunity in the recommendations of the plague conference and created the North Manchurian Plague Prevention Service in the spring of 1912. Interestingly, the Chinese government saw customs revenues as a legitimate way to fund hospitals and, subsequently, the Plague Prevention Service. Customs receipts, however, were under the control of the collected diplomatic representatives of foreign governments in Peking. This odd arrangement was a consequence of the Boxer Rebellion of 1899: the indemnities and foreign loans owed the powers were to be paid from customs duties, and to ensure equitable and reliable payments, they were administered by the diplomatic body in Peking. Initially, the foreigners refused to allocate funds for the very purpose that their representatives had recommended the year before. The argument against such spending was that there was no evidence of plague that year, and no reasonable prediction that it would return. The very notion of prevention was dismissed as a waste of money.[50] Eventually Wu Lien-Teh managed to enlist Sir Francis Aglen, the British inspector general of Chinese Maritime Customs, to the Chinese cause and the sum of sixty thousand taels (about forty thousand dollars) was appropriated annually for the support of the Plague Prevention Service based in Harbin.[51]

The North Manchurian Plague Prevention Service has been recognized by both Chinese and Western observers as the beginning of public health in China.[52] It was highly Westernized, with a senior staff of ethnic Chinese who had been educated in Western medicine. Junior staff physicians were often graduates of Western medical schools in China. Later, because its responsibilities extended beyond its original mandate, the name was changed to the Manchurian Plague Prevention Service and then gave rise to the National Quarantine Service. Its work on plague, initially stemming from investigation of the 1910–1911 epidemic, made it a worldwide center of plague research. The Health Organization of the League of Nations published Wu's *Treatise on Pneumonic Plague* in 1926, which was superseded as the standard plague reference only by the 1954 WHO monograph *Plague*, by Robert Pollitzer, one of Wu's protégés at the Plague Prevention Service.[53] The Manchurian Plague Prevention Service functioned as the de facto public health organization for China until its demise 1931 in response to the Japanese occupation of Manchuria. Its successor, the National Quarantine Service, headquartered in Shanghai and under Wu's directorship, a national public health organization, was again ended by Japanese aggression in China in 1937.

The plague was a singular event in the genesis of Western medicine in China, but beyond its impact on public health, it provided an important focus for international conflicts, diplomacy, and intrigue in Northeast Asia in the early twentieth century. As a regional threat demanding attention, the plague gave Russia, Japan, China, and the United States new opportunities to test and refine their evolving diplomatic and geopolitical strategies in the emerging postcolonial world.

CHAPTER FIVE

The Plague's Origin: Disease Ecology

MANCHUS AND MARMOTS: CULTURE AND NATURE

Manchuria in 1910 was a land of contrasts: a site of international rivalry and commercial competition, a region of problematic relationship to the future of the Chinese empire, and a place of contrasting cultures and traditional practices. In such a context the plague epidemic and its wider ramifications can be best understood against a background of local particulars. For many Chinese, Manchuria represented a distant land, a frontier culturally, politically, and geographically. The land of the Manchus was home to a people considered distinctly foreign and, as Crossley described, objects of xenophobic hostility by the majority Han population.[1] Suddenly, however, Manchuria was a site of global interest, a region of considerable economic importance, a land of strange customs and products, a geographic frontier with Russia and a region of conflict with Japan. Of particular relevance to the spread of plague was the burgeoning Manchurian fur trade at the end of the nineteenth century.

THE CHINESE FRONTIER

Manchu culture and customs differed from those of the Chinese in ways obvious even to the casual foreign observer: the dress, particularly for women, was distinctly different; Manchu women did not submit to the Chinese practice of foot binding, wearing, instead, thick-soled shoes, often four to six inches high, which accentuated their already tall carriage. They wore long, loose gowns similar to those of Manchu men and kept their hair in a distinctive coiffure.[2] The long history of the Qing government was infused with a more or less consistent theme of distinction and veneration of Manchu culture, as befitted its ancestral, non-Chinese origins. The very concept of "Manchuria" was developed by the Qing in the eighteenth century as a concept to buffer China from its northern neighbors, the Russians.[3] Manchu culture, however, proved less resilient and stable than that of the other border peoples, the Mongols. Although Mongol identity and language persisted, by the early twentieth century, Manchu as a language was fading, and many Manchus had assimilated, in spite of the waves of racism and nationalism on the part of the Han majority in China. Manchuria in 1911, however, was still seen as a safe and secure refuge for persecuted Manchus living in other parts of China.[4]

The new railways in Manchuria immediately brought an influx of Chinese immigrants, both permanent and transient, many from Shandong province, only a boat ride across the Gulf of Pechili. Starting in Dairen, these immigrants moved northward and sought work in the coal and iron mines of Manchuria, on farms, and in the fur trade of the frontier regions. In the city of Feng t'ien (the Chinese quarter of Mukden) in 1906, Frank Leeming estimated that the carting of goods employed 20 percent of the workforce and was second only to domestic service, the major occupation of the working class.[5] In Feng t'ien of 1906, there were about twice as many men as women, again suggesting that transient, migratory workers with families left behind elsewhere made use of the railway to seek new jobs and new opportunities.

The population of Manchuria in 1910 was about 12.5 million, most of whom resided outside of the few large cities.[6] The major urban areas included the old Manchu capital of Feng t'ien (Mukden), a city of 180,000 in 1906; Harbin, the railway city developed by Russia between 1896 and 1905, with a populace in the first decade of the twentieth century of about 40,000; Dairen, the southern terminus of the railway system on the Gulf of Pechili, with an estimated population of 40,000; and nearby Port Arthur, a smaller but important seaport of 14,000 inhabitants.[7]

By the end of the first decade of the twentieth century, traditional Manchu culture was under attack in the north by the increasing Russianization of the regions along the Russian-owned Chinese Eastern Railroad. The northern city of Harbin was a center of Russian culture and influence. In the south, the foreign influence was Japanese. Since acquiring the new Russian commercial port city of Dalny (renamed Dairen) following the Russo-Japanese War, Japan was importing a thoroughly modern Japanese culture all across the south of Manchuria. It was only in the central region, around the traditional Manchu capital city of Mukden, that these two clashing foreign interests still allowed Chinese and Manchu culture to exist in relative peace.

In the villages and towns along the Chinese frontier with Russia, life was rough and ready, far from the authority of either Peking or St. Petersburg. In Manchouli, the small Chinese town at the terminus of the Chinese Eastern Railway, ten miles east of the Siberian border, there were about two hundred Russian houses confined to the railway district, and the normal population consisted of about five thousand Russians and two thousand Chinese. During the marmot-hunting season, however, the Chinese population swelled to about ten thousand. Photographs of Manchouli from 1910 show a flat, treeless landscape with low, plain single-story buildings lined up along wide, unpaved roads; the hostile climate was hot and dusty in summer and bitter cold in winter, with scant snow cover. It even lacked the usual riverside location of major trading towns. Its border location on the main railway route across Central Asia gave Manchouli a strategic importance far beyond its natural attractions. The one hotel for travelers has remained infamous for more than a century.

The contrast between urban and rural life was typical of colonial culture. Western architecture and city development had invaded Asia in the mid–nineteenth century, typified by the wide French boulevards of Saigon, the Greek revival buildings of the Bund in Shanghai, the Yamato Hotels along the South Manchuria Railway, and the ornate Orthodox churches in Harbin. Beyond these few focal points of European influence, however, Manchuria was traditional and nearly untouched by the growing ambitions of the Great Powers.

What is now called infrastructure was nearly nonexistent outside the few major urban centers: "The roads in Manchuria are bad, being little more than tracks, more or less defined, between town and town."[8] The scarcity of building stone in Manchuria precluded the construction of more permanent avenues of transport. In the rainy season, these tracks, often below the level of the surrounding land, became muddy quagmires. One visitor reported seeing a mule drown in the flooded roadway. In winter, however, when frozen solid, these roads were heavy with traffic of two-wheeled carts. "These vehicles, each carrying from 1 1/2 to 3 1/2 tons and drawn by as many as eight or nine mules, travel in convoys sometimes half a mile in length, bearing a miscellaneous freight of native and foreign produce."[9] In addition, the abundant waterways provided efficient barge transportation in summer and served as roadways for cart traffic when frozen in winter.

Travelogues of the time described the exoticism of Manchuria, sometimes strange even to those familiar with traditional China. Even gory photographs of execution day, showing piles of severed heads of "bandits," were included in these accounts for armchair adventurers.[10] On a visit to Tsitsithar (Qiqihar), a medium-sized town in northern Manchuria, in the spring of 1911, the adventurer Richardson Wright not only provided a vivid description of the public holiday devoted to the execution of criminals but gave a colorful, and unabashedly Eurocentric, account of city street life:

> At one of the booths in the main bazaar of Tsitsitcar [*sic*] they sell strips of shining brown, glutinous, ribbon sea weed. At another sat a pair of letter writers. . . . Over there squats a cobbler with his gear spread out in the dust. The cobblers of Tsitsitcar, like the letter writers, the barbers, the doctors and pretty much everyone else, work in the open street. The doctors work in teams of two. They rig up a tent furnished with chairs and a counter spread with bushels of trash, love potions, charms, incantations, neck ornaments to scare away devils, potato bugs and the plague, a dozen dirty little bottles of simple medicaments, glycerine, iodine, spirits of nitre, stuff in common demand in the drug store. Pinned to the side of the tent are gruesome colored native anatomical charts. Up comes a patient. The doctor pushes him into a chair and then and there hears his tale of woe or dresses his wound or does anything else that has to be done, all of it without the least privacy. The patient returns a stolid glare to the gaping crowd around and does not seem to object to them in the slightest degree.[11]

As the ancestral home of the Qing rulers, Manchuria was a place of importance in maintaining the legitimacy of Manchu supremacy and of Manchu power. The Qing government continued to support Manchu garrisons of supporters in China at increasing cost to the imperial treasury well into the nineteenth century and to require the use of the Manchu language as a medium for communication of state secrets. Edicts requiring the Qing officials to be proficient in Manchu (a non-Chinese language written in a derivative of Mongol script) were repetitive and increasingly ineffective. The Qing had struggled since its inception in 1644 to find the appropriate relationship between Manchuria and the rest of China. Often its policies revolved around immigration schemes, not only encouraging Chinese, especially from nearby provinces, to move to Manchuria to increase agricultural production as well as to dilute local Manchu power, but also using it as a place of exile for troublesome Manchu dependents (so-called Bannermen).[12] Being far from the center of imperial power in Peking, and under the authority of an official variously called viceroy, governor-general, or governor, it was in a way the "Wild West of China."

In 1899, as a harbinger of things to come, plague in its bubonic form became epidemic in the southern regions of China, most notably centered in Hong Kong.[13] In July of that year, the first recorded case in the north was noted by a Western physician in Newchwang in a village just outside the city walls. It was believed to have been imported from the raging Hong Kong epidemic. There was a busy commercial traffic between Hong Kong and Swatow in the south and the port of Newchwang in the northeast of China. Although the epidemic in Manchuria took hold immediately, it was two months and two thousand deaths later before the Chinese government took action. A Sanitary Board was established in Newchwang, plague hospitals and a plague cemetery were set up, and rudimentary elements of quarantine were established. The board engaged fifteen Japanese physicians and a Japanese sanitary engineer, who were joined by three volunteer Russian physicians. The approach to this epidemic was based on the best science of the period, namely, sanitation and quarantine of cases, although the board was expressly forbidden by the Chinese government from instituting any mandatory regulations.[14] Interestingly, the head of the Sanitary Board, Sir Alexander Hosie, was able to use this early epidemic to conduct basic investigations into the nature of plague. He determined, in some detail, the environmental conditions of temperature, humidity, and nutrition for survival of the newly discovered plague bacillus.[15] This early epidemic reached its peak in the summer of 1899, and by December it was over. The disease was reported to be almost entirely confined to the Chinese population, with only a few deaths among the foreign residents noted.

THE RUSSIAN PRESENCE

Russian influence and presence in the valley of the Amur River (Heilung Jiang) dated from at least the sixteenth century, and by the seventeenth century the Qing found it useful to construct the concept of "Manchuria" as the ancestral land of its origin to solidify its claims and to mobilize support in these ongoing territorial disputes with the Romanov Empire.[16] The impetus for the Treaty of Nerchinsk in 1689 was the need to stabilize and eliminate the repeated frontier conflicts between the peoples of Qing China, mainly Mongolians and Manchus, and the populations under the sovereignty of Russia along the Amur River region. Even so, this border region was still contested well into twentieth century. Not only were there many Russians doing business and trading back and forth across the border, but the influx of Russian immigrants was turning some of the towns on the Chinese side into de facto Russian enclaves. The main instrument of this colonization in modern times was the railroad. As the main overland gateway between Russia and China since the coming of the railroad, towns such as Irgun on the Russian side and Manchouli on the Chinese side took on added importance beyond their traditional role as transportation depots along the Amur and its collateral water routes.

The completion of the Russian railway route, shortcutting, as it were, across Manchuria from Manchouli at the Russia-China border on the west to Vladivostok on the east, via Tsitsihar and Harbin in Manchuria, provided a Russian corridor cutting a swath across the region and firmly implanting Russian colonial influence in northern China. Harbin, as the headquarters for the Russian railway enterprise in China (incongruously named the Chinese Eastern Railway), became, in the course of a few years, a thriving Russian city on Chinese soil. As in South Manchuria where the South Manchuria Railway was an instrument of Japanese colonial policy, so in North Manchuria, the Chinese Eastern Railway administration was intimately connected with the Imperial Russian government. The overlap of the military, civil, and economic activities was extensive, and probably even more complex and convoluted than in the Japanese case in the south.

Of particular interest for the present discussion are the various public health and medical policies and practices established in the Russian-controlled regions of Manchuria. In addition to hospitals and medical services for the employees of the Chinese Eastern Railway and the Russian population in these colonies, the medical authorities often had responsibilities for some basic public health activities such as monitoring for epidemic diseases and advising the government and railroad officials on sanitation, quarantine, and related matters.

A sketchy and incomplete picture of the Russian medical presence in the towns along the railway and extending out into the Manchurian countryside can be pieced together from scattered sources. The general view that emerges is of a surprisingly sophisticated level of medical care and staffing. The Russian railway company maintained physicians at Manchouli as well as at other places along the Chinese Eastern Railway, not only to provide the usual medical services to the Russian population but also to help enforce quarantines.

THE JAPANESE PRESENCE

It was along the southern seacoast of Manchuria and along the central railway corridor of the South Manchuria Railway Company that the Japanese influence was most pronounced. The key port cities of Newchwang, Port Arthur, and Dairen were the "doors" for trade as well as military action in Manchuria, and as such were the key prizes won by Japan from Russia after the defeat of the latter in the Russo-Japanese War (1904–1905). While Newchwang and Port Arthur were existing Manchurian cities, Dairen was an entirely new city, originally laid out and planned by the Russians to be their major commercial, ice-free port to complement the military harbor and installation at nearby Port Arthur, only fourteen miles along the coast. The original impetus for the construction of an entirely new port in South Manchuria came from the Russian military, which objected to the commingling of the "open" commercial and "strategic" military uses of the harbor at Port Arthur. In addition, Sergei Witte, the Russian finance minister, believed that the railway and harbor enterprises should be integrated, modeled after the success of the Canadian Pacific Railway and the port of Vancouver. Dairen soon became a major locus for the importation of Chinese tea into Russia (half of Russia's tea in 1903) as well as the outlet for Manchurian agricultural produce.[17]

Originally named Dalny (The Faraway Place) and planned by Russia in the then-popular international "garden city" form, this incipient "Paris of the Far East" was in disrepair and incomplete by the time it fell into Japanese hands after the war. Japan inherited a nearly blank slate and proceeded to develop a fully modern city, a showcase with wide boulevards, hospitals, hotels, schools, and other infrastructure unlike any other Chinese city.[18] As the headquarters and eventual terminus of the South Manchuria Railway, it was a key site for both commercial and military activity.

The northern terminus of the South Manchuria Railway was in Ch'ang ch'un, an old Manchurian town some seventy miles northeast of Mukden. At Ch'ang ch'un the rail gauge changed, and the railway continued on to Harbin as the Russian-owned Chinese Eastern Railway. A crucial development by the Japanese was the exploitation of rich coal fields at Fushun and Yentai, located on short rail spurs just outside of Mukden. A side branch of the South Manchuria Railway ran from Mukden to the Korean border at Antung, thereby providing Japan with rail access to its newly acquired interests in Korea as well. Thus, the traditional Manchu seat at Mukden, too, would gradually feel the changes being pushed on China by the Japanese colonial enterprise.

THE FUR TRADE

One attraction for the men of Shantung from across the Gulf of Pechili was the lucrative fur trade of Manchuria. Two sorts of fur

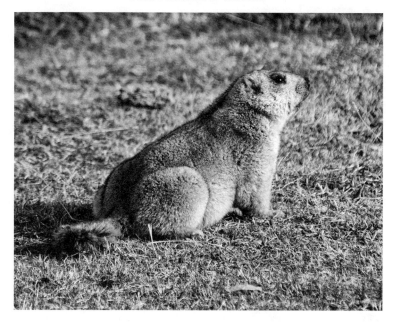

Figure 12. Mongolian marmot (*Marmota sibirica*).
(Reproduced with permission of David Blank)

made up the bulk of Manchurian fur exports: that of dogs, specifically raised for their pelts, and that of the wild rodent of the steppes
known as the Mongolian marmot (fig. 12). It was the latter that
provided new opportunities for the wandering immigrant trappers from the south. These common burrowing rodents had been
a staple in the diet of the Mongolian and northern Manchurian
peoples at least since the thirteenth century, when they were described in Western accounts by Marco Polo (ca. 1254–1324) and
William of Rubruck (ca. 1220–1293).[19] As Polo noted, "They [the
native peoples] live on meat and milk and game and on Pharaoh's
rats [marmots], which are abundant everywhere in the steppes"
and "on which they live all summer, since they are creatures of

some size." Friar William noted that marmots hibernate in winter in large burrows: "They have also certain little beasts called by them sogur [marmots], which lie in a cave twenty or thirty of them together, all the whole winter sleeping for the space of six months. These they take in great abundance." Modern culinary sources describe the preparation of marmot as following the traditional method of filling the body with red-hot stones and then grilling to make a dish called "bodok."[20] It was this little animal that would play several important roles in bringing the devastation of plague to Manchuria.

The Mongolian marmot (*Marmota sibirica*) is a larger relative of the common yellow-bellied marmot (*M. flaviventris*) and the woodchuck (*M. monax*) seen in North America and is a common inhabitant of the high steppes of Mongolia and Manchuria. These animals are active in the summer and mature in about three years. They have relatively small litters, about three to four pups, yet until recently the populations seemed quite stable.[21] The name for this animal in Russian is *tarbagan*, in Mongolian, *tarvaga*, and in Chinese, *hàn-tă* (dry-land otter). The steppes of Central Asia and Northeast China provide the open grazing land for the nomadic peoples who have traditionally hunted marmots for both food and clothing. By the nineteenth century, however, when sedentary agriculture and herding had replaced nomadism to a large extent, marmot hunting was mainly a subsistence activity of the poor. Traditionally, the fat-rich marmot provided high-calorie food as well as several folk medicines.[22]

Mongolian marmot fur is somewhat coarse, light yellow-brown in color, and although it was long used for local clothing, it was not considered a valuable fur until the early twentieth century. The 1911 edition of the *Encyclopaedia Britannica* described it derisively: "It should always be a cheap fur, having so few good

qualities to recommend it."[23] In the 1890s, however, the burgeoning German chemical industry had a big impact on the
marmot hunters in faraway Manchuria. The new aniline dyes of
the organic chemist allowed furriers in Leipzig and Vienna to
color marmot fur in ways that mimicked sable, otter, and mink,
all expensive and highly prized furs. The Berlin Aniline Company marketed a series of aromatic amine dyes for fur under the
generic name of "Ursols."[24] They were introduced in Leipsig in
about 1898 and in England a year later. The dyeing of marmot fur
became a major activity of both Leipsig and English dyers at that
time.[25] Prior to the introduction of these synthetic dyes, wood-
based dyes, which required much skill and experience to use, were
the only dyes available. The advent of the Ursols, however, "led to
a great increase in the number of fur dyers, most of whom knew
practically nothing about the fur-dyeing business, and the result was anticipated. The cost of dying Marmots was first about
9d. [pence] to 1s. [shilling] each, but as soon as the smaller dyers
entered into competition they cut the prices, which eventually fell
to 7d., 6d., and finally 3d."[26]

The Viennese furriers developed a method for dyeing fur
garments after the article was finished so that a perfectly sym-
metrical shading and striping could be obtained without the need
for laboriously matching many naturally colored small pelts.[27]
As an example of the demand for marmot fur, the London fur
market for 1905–1906 reported sales of 1.6 million marmot pelts
compared to only 80,000 beaver skins and were exceeded only by
squirrel, possum, muskrat, and kid pelts.[28] These marmot pelts
went for between 9 pence and 2 shilling, 6 pence each.[29]

The markets of Asia, too, were active in marmot fur. Mongolian records of exports to Russia indicate that only thirty thousand
marmot pelts were exported in 1865; by 1892 that number had

risen to 1.4 million, and during 1906–1910 to 13 million, a four-hundredfold increase. Since these data are limited to Russian exports and do not include exports to other countries, they certainly do not reflect the full scope of the marmot hunting craze.[30]

There were several methods for hunting marmots. Most hunting techniques relied on the belief that the marmot is an intensely curious animal and can be approached by the hunter if its attention can be focused on some intriguing action or device. One traditional method was to employ a well-trained hunting dog that would attract the attention of the marmot by acting like a natural predator. Rather than run for cover, the animal would remain above ground in a frozen posture while watching the stealthy approach of the dog. The hunter could then approach close enough to shoot the animal, traditionally with a bow and arrow, but in modern times with a rifle. A more colorful method was used by a hunter without a trained marmot dog. The traditional hunter wore an unusual costume: white pants, white jacket and a hat with hare-like ears that often stood straight up in the air (fig. 13). He employed a tassel six to eight inches long, called a *daluur*, made from a white horse or yak tail attached to a small wooden handle. The hunter shook the *daluur*, and, if all went well, the marmot became excited and emitted its characteristic warning call but did not hide. The hunter would then zigzag toward his prey, taking tiny steps; he stooped down so that the ears on his hat stood out against the sky. When he was within ninety to one hundred feet of the animal, he would drop on all fours. If the marmot had stopped calling, the hunter would wag his head to make the white ears wiggle so as to further excite the marmot. This hunting behavior has been interpreted as an imitation of the marmot's natural canine predator, the wolf, which elicits the prolonged calling and presumably its distraction.

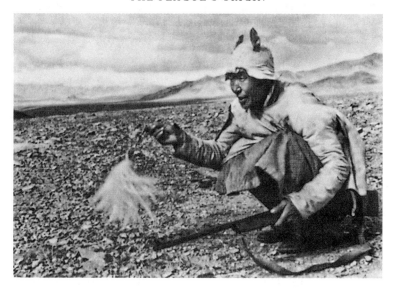

Figure 13. A marmot hunter. (Photograph by Dugarsham
Tserennadmid; courtesy of Enrico Mascelloni)

With the influx of Chinese from Shantung, brought by
the new railway, organized teams of Russians and Chinese were
hired by rich fur merchants and equipped with the necessities for
marmot hunting. These teams, especially the newly arrived Chinese, did not use the traditional methods, but resorted to snares
set at the entrances of the marmot burrows as well as digging out
the burrows in search of injured or even sick animals.[31] There were
both spring and fall hunting seasons. The spring season ran from
mid-March to the end of May, and the fall season from late August to mid-October. Since pelts harvested in the fall were considered of higher quality and brought higher prices, the fall hunting
season was more popular, and the 1910 fall marmot hunt was
no exception. Anatole S. Loukashkin (1902–1988), the Russian
marmot authority, estimated that in 1909–1911 there were more

than twelve thousand hunters in organized teams in northern Manchuria.[32] In addition to these organized groups, there were also many freelance itinerant hunters. This newer mode of aggressive hunting, driven by the rise in world demand for marmot fur, would eventually lead to the decimation of the marmot colonies in Manchuria by the mid-1920s.[33]

The Mongolian marmot warning call is reported to sound like the Chinese words *pu p'a* (pinyin, bù pà, no fear), which the hunter took as the sign that the animal was healthy. Hunters also professed to be able to identify diseased marmots by making an incision on the paw; if it bled freely, the animal was judged healthy. Often, however, the skins of sick marmots were sold even though such animals were rejected as food.

The traditional marmot hunting methods have been interpreted by some researchers as aimed at avoiding animals infected with plague. Even late-nineteenth-century accounts of tarbagan hunting describe the important role of this ubiquitous rodent in the lives of the population of Transbaikalia and Mongolia.[34] The animal was valued for its meat, its pelt, and its abundant fat, used both for greasing leather objects and for lighting. This fat was sold by the barrelful in the Siberian towns of Nerchinsk and Stretensk. Russian observers reported a periodic epizootic disease that was well recognized by the natives and called by the Russian name *chyma*, meaning "plague" (in Russian *chyma* is used for the disease caused by *Y. pestis*, but it has a wider use in the vernacular, including cattle plague and Siberian plague, which is anthrax).[35] The symptoms of this disease in the marmots are described as follows: "The animal becomes languid, and ceases to bark; its gait is unsteady, and under one shoulder there sometimes appears a reddish, tense swelling; if far from its hole the animal fails to find it and easily falls prey to its foes. . . . They [the Buriats] have another test to determine whether the animal is diseased or not. They cut into the sole of one paw, and if they find the blood coagulated they consider the animal diseased and give it to the dogs to eat. It is an interesting fact that neither dogs nor wolves—the latter of which eat up the tarbagans in immense numbers—ever contract the disease." The commentator, Frank G. Clemow, a British expert on exotic diseases, speculated that the taste of wolves for sick marmots may explain "the comparative rarity with which the disease is transmitted to humans."[36] The disease could, however, cause fatal disease in humans, and he describes several local outbreaks in Transbaikalia and in Mongolia that occurred in families occupied in tarbagan hunting, skinning, or otherwise closely associated with this animal. These local accounts all report rapid onset and nearly 100 percent mortality among those afflicted. Taken together, these early reports show that local knowledge included understanding of both the marmot epizootics as well its danger to humans. The rather ritualized hunting may have had the effect of taking only healthy animals. Such methods could have originated in a combination of animal shamanism or other cultural practices with empirical observations of the recurrent epizootics.[37]

A main center for marmot hunting is in the northern regions of Manchuria along the Heilongjiang (Amur River). Here the northern taiga meets the mountain steppes and gives way in the south to open plains. The climate is dry, and the seasonal changes are extreme. Marmot hunters in the first decade of the twentieth century had a hard life. One metropolitan Chinese observed: "Often they fail to get anything to eat or to drink. Consequently they eat the flesh of the marmot and drink water squeezed out of a towel which has been left on the grass during the night to catch the dew. Hunters under such circumstances are naturally weakened and predisposed to any infection. On their arrival at Dawoolya,

Manchouli, or other towns they are packed in rooms somewhat like sardines in a box and thus easily contract and spread plague."[38]

Since Manchouli was one of the principle marmot fur trading centers, such a seasonal influx of hunters and fur traders overwhelmed the available housing. One contemporary observer noted: "I made some observations on the types of dwellings occupied by these hunters when they return from their work. They are built of strong timber laid out in small blocks of one story in height. Into each compartment from twenty to forty bunks arranged in three or four tiers may be seen. The windows are seldom if ever opened, and when the rooms are crowded during the hunting season, the smell emanating from the occupants and from the raw skins which they often bring with them is not pleasant, and probably paves the way for infection in epidemic form."[39]

The pelts, usually removed from the animals in the field immediately upon trapping the marmots, were dried, bundled into bales of 1,000 to 1,780 skins, subjected to disinfection by the Chinese Eastern Railway (beginning in 1911), and then exported to the main markets in England, the United States, Russia, and Germany.[40] Little did the migrant gangs of marmot trappers realize that the seemingly unlimited bounty of these little animals would also turn out to be the source of death and devastation, brought on by disruption in the traditional hunting patterns, which maintained the fragile ecology of endemic plague.

PLAGUE RESERVOIRS AND HISTORY

Historians exhibit a fascination with origin stories that is certainly natural to their calling. This is especially the case for epidemic disease. Indeed, the "historical method" is central to the scientific approaches of the epidemiologist as well. Plague origins are no exception, and the stories told range from speculative to poetic. The origin of the Manchurian plague has been discussed by several authors, including Wu Lien-Teh, one of the key participants in dealing with the epidemic, and several respected historians. Uncertainties have been recognized: first, since investigation of the earliest cases was not carried out, only sketchy accounts of the initial deaths are available, and second, the role of the marmot as the origin of this specific epidemic is only circumstantial.

In addition to examining origin stories, some historically minded physicians and scientists often ask, "Is this disease the same disease that we know today?" or sometimes more simply, "Was it *really* the plague?" There are two reactions to such questions. One response is, "Does it matter?" Does it matter that we identify the Plague of Athens with some currently known disease, or is it enough to know what the Athenians made of it, what effects it had on their world, and what subsequent peoples thought about it? Alternately, another response asks, What additional historical questions can we ask about the epidemic if we can apply modern knowledge of the disease to the historical context? Thus, the project of "retrospective diagnosis" has its advocates as well as its detractors.[41] It is important to note, however, that in the case of the great Manchurian plague, we are quite confident in our diagnosis: there is no doubt that the Manchurian population was made sick by infection with *Y. pestis*. Whether this organism was the same one that was involved in earlier epidemics, say the Black Death or the Plague of Justinian, may be an interesting question, but it is irrelevant to understanding the cause of the Manchurian plague, in spite of some attempts to do so.[42]

Science does, however, offer insights that bear on our understanding of the history, evolution, and ecology of plague as an organism and as an affliction of humans and of animals. Historians have properly questioned origin stories and retrospective diagnoses, and plague, especially the fourteenth-century epidemic later known as the Black Death, has attracted almost as much attention as the Plague of Athens, as described by Thucydides. Traditionally, the Black Death has been held to be an epidemic associated with *Y. pestis*, although revisionist history, based on questions of symptomatology, rat populations, and epidemiological considerations, has questioned *Y. pestis* as the real cause of this plague (and some others). These hypotheses, however, have recently been effectively overturned by biological evidence that is unequivocal and shows that the Black Death was, indeed, an epidemic of *Y. pestis*.[43] DNA samples from multiple grave sites from the time of this epidemic consistently yield evidence of a unique and specific variant of *Y. pestis* in the very regions where the plague's devastation was most extensive.

One of the first attempts to use modern bacteriological science to supplement the global historical account of plague was Devignat's proposal in 1951 that bacteriological classification of the subgroups of the plague bacillus, called biovars (abbreviated bv.), could be used to trace outbreaks, because these biovars seem to be geographically specific.[44] Thus, he identified three biovars: *orientalis*, which was the cause of the modern or third global pandemic; *antiqua*, which is confined to Central and Northeast Asia as well as Central Africa and which he speculated caused the ancient plagues of history, the Plague of Justinian in the sixth century, for example; and *mediaevalis*, found in the steppes of Russia and which he suggested was the biovar that caused the great medieval or second pandemic represented by the Black Death of the mid–fourteenth century. These biovars of *Y. pestis* were initially characterized by their cultural characteristics—that is, the requirements each type showed for growth in cultures on petri dishes in the laboratory. For example, *orientalis* could not grow with just glycerin as a source of carbohydrate for energy, whereas *antiqua* could.

Devignat's proposal led to serious study by bacteriologists who immediately appreciated the refinement of *Y. pestis* classification, but it was perhaps too general and did not account for unusual variants to allow for stringent testing of historical hypotheses. Recently, however, the determination of the entire DNA sequence of several *Yersinia* species together with the analysis of hundreds of isolates for specific genetic sequences has allowed scientists to construct an unambiguous family tree of global *Y. pestis* variants.[45] This new knowledge can be used to examine several recent historical accounts of plague epidemics.

The recent genomic studies summarized by Morelli et al. examined nearly a thousand isolates of *Y. pestis* from different geographic regions.[46] Two major conclusions of this analysis are that *Y. pestis* evolved between fifteen hundred and twenty thousand years ago in China, from an ancestral *Yersinia* species called *Yersinia pseudotuberculosis*, and that an unambiguous phylogenetic tree with a single origin can relate all the isolates of *Y. pestis* to each other. *Y. pseudotuberculosis* is a bacterium that causes a usually self-limited intestinal infection in humans and animals.[47] In rare instances, however, it can invade the bloodstream, where it leads to a severe and often fatal septicemia. In the evolution of *pseudotuberculosis* to *pestis*, there has been acquisition of genes, both chromosomal and on virulence plasmids, that confer the ability to infect and be transmitted by fleas as well as the ability to easily invade the bloodstream. Thus, this evolution involved changes in both the vector ecology as well as the pathophysiological distribution in the host body. In addition to the three classical biovars of *pestis*, however, a recently identified biovar named *microtus* (the genus of many voles) has been found in Central Asia and Inner Mongolia, with the Siberian marmot as its principal reservoir.[48] This biovar is interesting in that its pathogenicity seems to be limited to rodents, and it is avirulent in humans.

In trying to correlate biovars of *Y. pestis* with the origins and spread (called "radiations" by evolutionary biologists) with historical records, Achtman and his colleagues show that the New World isolates all originated from the Hong Kong epidemic of 1894–1895, as suggested earlier on circumstantial evidence by writers such as Eschenberg, Benedict, and others.[49] Further, these molecular data strongly support the belief that the initial emergence of *Y. pestis* from *Y. pseudotuberculosis* occurred in Central Asia or China, a region where the marmot has been a dominant species for centuries. Li et al. have identified seven of the fifteen plague foci in present-day China as being associated with marmots.[50]

With these new data in hand, we can now seek more detail as to the origin of the great Manchurian plague. Since this plague first appeared in the border regions between Manchuria and Transbaikalia, in the very regions where *antiqua* biovars still exist, and where the offshoot animal bv. *microtus* still is endemic in the marmot population, it is most unlikely that the radiation of *orientalis* biovar from the epidemic in Hong Kong was involved. While we do not (yet) have DNA sequence analysis of any samples directly connected to the Manchurian plague, or even from northwestern Manchuria (although it is possible that samples from graves of victims might still be informative), the most parsimonious interpretation is that of simple direct spread from its ancestral home in Central Asia eastward into Mongolia and Manchuria.[51] The few data on current biovars from Northeast China support this independent migration hypothesis. Of the eight

Y. pestis samples from Northeast China that have been analyzed by genomic DNA sequencing and reported in the literature, six were bv. *antiqua* and two were bv. *mediaevalis*.[52] Phylogenetically, these particular strains of these biovars are very early offshoots (so-called branch 2) of the main (root) stem of the evolutionary tree from *Y. pseudotuberculosis*, a fact that indicates their likely indigenous Central Asian ancestry rather than a descent from later radiations via the Yunnan–Hong Kong branch that is represented by bv. *orientalis*.[53]

NICHES: CULTURAL AND BIOLOGICAL

Epidemic disease is one manifestation of a change in ecological niche. As an infectious agent adapts, new balances must be struck with respect to both host and parasite, and alternatively, as a host changes, new selections often drive new adaptations in microbes. We have seen, in the case of the Great Plague in Manchuria, that new populations, new technologies, and new politics all contributed to the spread of *Y. pestis* and the disruption of the more or less stable equilibrium that existed in the traditional Asian communities of humans and marmots. Epidemics can result from newly virulent strains, but probably more often, it is the opening of new niches by human actions that provides new opportunities for disease expansions. What was the cause of the Great Plague? Simply the "plague bacillus"? Ignorant marmot hunters? Chemists in Leipsig? Railway moguls in Russia and Japan? Insufficient public health measures? Paralyzed political systems? The answer: all of the above.

CHAPTER SIX

Plague and Politics

GEOPOLITICAL RIVALRIES IN MANCHURIA

While national rivalries and geopolitical concerns often surfaced in the day-to-day accounts of the plague itself and even more so in the events connected with the international plague conference in Mukden, the diplomatic record of the Manchurian plague is rich with examples of subtle and not so subtle political maneuvers by the governments concerned with their interests in Manchuria as well as the larger East Asian sphere.

The most obvious and public competitors in Manchuria were Russia and Japan, but the French, British, Germans, and Americans all had interests there as well. China, although weak in almost every way possible, was desperately employing every diplomatic and political asset it could muster to balance the Great Powers to its own advantage. While Russia was backed by French and, to some extent, German interests, Japan was supported by Great Britain as a counterbalance against the Russians. The United States, without the traditional alliances of the European powers, opted for a policy of neutrality, optimistically framed in terms of Hay's Open Door Policy. But how did these international macro-policies play out on Manchurian soil in the midst of one of the worst plague epidemics in history?

JAPAN IN MANCHURIA AND KOREA

Japan had the most comprehensive, consistent, and determined policy toward Manchuria, which led to total occupation, the establishment of the puppet state of Manchukuo in 1932, and the tragedy of World War II in Asia. From 1603 until 1867, Japan had been ruled by military warlords (*shogun*, a military title more or less equivalent to "generalissimo") of the Tokugawa clan. Partly spurred on by the challenge to Japanese isolationism from the forced "opening" of Japan to foreign trade by the American fleet under Commodore Matthew Perry in 1853, the Tokugawa Shogun ceded power to the Japanese emperor, previously an impotent figurehead. The young supporters of the new emperor Meiji and this "restoration" of imperial rule in 1868 quickly undertook to modernize Japan along Western lines, most notably in terms of military modernization. Studies in Western language, culture, and especially science and technology were encouraged and became instruments of state policy.

Military modernization and Western learning nurtured national pride among the Japanese and led to their identification as "white Asians"—that is, Asians, but on a par with Europeans in their self-perceived social and cultural standing.[1] Japan's belief in its destiny to be the leader of what eventually became a Pan-Asian movement in World War II contributed to its expansionist policies in both Korea and, a bit later, in Manchuria.

Increasingly, during the nineteenth century Korea was the

focus of international rivalry between China and Japan, leading ultimately to the Sino-Japanese War in 1894–1895. While Korea did not seem overtly involved in the Great Plague, its role in regional geopolitics set much of the context within which the plague evolved. Although Korea had been a traditional tributary state that recognized nominal Chinese authority, in 1876 Korea and Japan concluded a treaty, the first article of which stated that Korea was an independent state.[2] In 1882, however, the Chinese issued trade regulations relating to Korea which asserted that the Korean peninsula was a Chinese tributary state. In response to this renewed Chinese assertion of suzerainty, the Japanese stiffened their opposition to Chinese hegemony in Korea. As both China and Japan grew in strength, this contradictory situation in Korea provided the root cause for future trouble. Contending factions in the Korean court contributed to instability in Seoul, and when antiforeign disturbances broke out in 1882 with the loss of several Japanese lives, there was a clamor for war on the part of some militarists in Japan. After hurried diplomatic efforts, both the Chinese and Japanese ended up with troops stationed in Seoul. Although a later agreement between Japan and China led to withdrawal of most of the troops, in 1894 a rebellion among antiforeign elements in Korea led to the dispatch of Chinese troops to Korea, the stated purpose of which was, in the words of the Chinese notification to the Japanese, "to restore the peace of our tributary state." Japan rejected such language and sent troops as well. The Korean king asked, without success, that both parties leave the country, but Japan, believing that official corruption was the root cause of the rebellion, unilaterally occupied the palace and pressured the Koreans to abrogate their treaty with China and request that the Japanese expel the Chinese. With the Japanese sinking of a Chinese transport ship in late July 1894, China declared war on Japan, which reciprocated the following day.

The war was a disaster for China, and the overwhelming victory by Japan by mid-March 1895 was a surprise to most observers and a humiliation to the Chinese. The ensuing negotiations and eventual peace treaty, which became known as the Treaty of Shimonoseki, the name of the Japanese city where it was signed, were so one-sided, severe, and humiliating to the Chinese that Russia, Germany, and France joined in pressuring Japan to ease its vengeance, in what became famous as the retrocession note of the Triple Intervention.

Even after Japan's agreement to milder treaty terms, Japan gained a substantial foothold in Manchuria with a long-term lease to the southern part of the Liaotung peninsula and the permanent control of Taiwan (Formosa). Both these expansionistic successes gave scope to Japanese ambitions to be the dominant geopolitical force in East Asia. And both of these new possessions were to be important in the Japanese strategies that played out in the Great Plague of 1910–1911. Thus, the configuration of Manchuria during the Great Plague was a direct consequence of the Korean policies of Japan and China.

Although the Treaty of Shimonoseki ended the active hostilities between Japan and China, the situation in Korea continued to deteriorate and on 22 August 1910 the ineffectual Korean government signed, without the approval of the Korean king, a treaty with Japan that gave Japan sovereignty in Korea. As recognized in the first of eight articles, the treaty stated: "His Majesty the Emperor of Korea makes the complete and permanent cession to His Majesty the Emperor of Japan of all rights of sovereignty over the whole of Korea." The annexation of Korea gave the Chinese even more evidence of Japan's expansionist designs in Northeast Asian, including Manchuria.

Japan's expansionist agenda was a concern, too, for the European powers and the United States. As early as 1907 President Theodore Roosevelt worried about war with Japan and even the possibility of a Japanese attack on the United States. German bets were clearly on the side of the Japanese. In confidential communications to the German chancellor in Berlin, Prince Bernhard von Bülow, the German ambassador in Washington, Baron Speck von Sternburg, wrote:

> Japan was doubtless aiming at control of the Pacific Ocean, extension of her territory southwards, and domination of China [marginalia by the German emperor: "Correct"]. . . . The President [Roosevelt] replied that with regard to the Navy an insoluble problem was before him—the face of a fortified harbor in the Far East as a base in the event of a great war with Japan. Even the best fleet must fail if after an engagement it had no such harbor to repair to. . . . The President mentioned the possibility of a Japanese invasion of the United States in the event of war. At the close of our conversation, after a long silence he spoke as follows: "If Japan invades America using powerful forces, our army will suffer a crushing blow. This lesson will produce a thorough military reorganization [marginalia by German emperor: 'That is no good in a war']; after this has been achieved, Japan's army will be annihilated if she has left it in America, and America will take her revenge [marginalia by German emperor: 'Very optimistic']."[3]

These concerns over Japanese expansionism were not unfounded speculations. Japanese actions and policies gave plenty of evidence of their reality. The Chinese model for hegemony over its neighbors had been refined over centuries and was based on the concept of tributary states that recognized China as the "Central Kingdom" but that retained semiautonomous status within that arrangement. Japan, on the other hand, based its expansion on the European colonial model. Occupation, economic domination and exploitation, and cultural change were all tactics to be used in its own concept of Japanese "manifest destiny." Taiwan, one of the spoils of the Sino-Japanese War, was an exemplary case study in Japanese colonialism for all to see.

Upon assuming control of Taiwan, the Japanese were faced with a rebellious and unruly population, much given to local uprisings.[4] Initially, Japanese policy in Taiwan was based on military efforts to suppress the local uprisings and "banditry," but soon it evolved into a more nuanced and sophisticated effort led by Gotō Shinpei.[5] The lessons learned in Taiwan would be directly applied a decade later in Manchuria. Gotō was a remarkable and talented individual, trained in Western medicine in Japan and public health in Germany (under Kitasato, no less), but a true statesman of Japan. Gotō was the protégé of General Kodama Gentarō (1852–1906), who became the military governor of Taiwan starting in 1898. Soon after their arrival in Taiwan, Gotō was appointed civil governor of Taiwan. Both Gotō and Kodama supported the idea that they were there to "govern" not to "conquer," and, not surprisingly, Gotō resorted to a biological metaphor to explain his colonial tactics: "In this era of scientific progress, the basic principle of colonization has to be built on biology. Then, what is the basis of biology? It is to encourage a scientific way of living, from which are derived the systems of industrial production, hygiene, education, transportation, and law enforcement. It is also to realize the principle of survival of the fittest in this competitive world."[6]

The main tactic that Gotō developed as the basis for Japanese colonial policy was scientific research into every aspect of the peoples and lands to be colonized. He noted that while the European colonial powers had sent out missionaries, explorers, and even scientific study teams to their colonies, Japan was new at this enterprise and could not simply force its customs and systems on the colonized peoples. He advocated wide-ranging study of local customs, legal systems, natural resources, economic developments, and the like. Indeed, in 1900 he established a research center in Taiwan to study local customs and traditions, and headed it himself. It had sections on legal research, economic research, and administrative research. By 1906 it had published voluminous reports on Taiwanese customs, religion, languages, ethics, psychology, handicrafts, and native living conditions.[7]

Gotō and his compatriots, however, did not see Taiwan as an isolated colonial responsibility, a troublesome spoil of the Sino-Japanese War, but rather as the springboard from which Japan could expand both economically and militarily into South China and the South Pacific and, eventually, into Northeast Asia as well. For Gotō, with his scientific background, research was the key to successful colonial policy. His policies were remarkably successful in Taiwan, and within seven years of his arrival in Taiwan, it had become economically independent of Japan.[8]

Japanese expansionism in Northeast Asia had focused on Manchuria and Korea for several decades, and at the close of the Russo-Japanese War, Japan again found itself faced with a potential problem in the form of the railways in its newly acquired Leased Territories in the Liaotung peninsula of Manchuria. The Japanese leadership was unsure about the future of the railways, the operation of which was complex, expensive, and difficult. The financial strain of the war had taken its toll in Japan, but to some, the railways represented one of the most valuable spoils of the costly war. Thus it was that the Japanese government established a government-owned company for the management of the railways in the Leased Territories. In June 1907 the South Manchuria

Railway Company came into existence by imperial ordinance. The Japanese Army in Manchuria, the de facto government after the end of the war, was headed by Gotō's mentor, General Kodama. Kodama invited Gotō to visit Manchuria and consult on the future of Japanese interests there. Kodama already saw the railways as an essential instrument of Japanese expansionism. In 1905 he suggested that "the most essential post-war policy in Manchuria is to carry out numerous secret projects under the pretext of running a railway company. The South Manchuria Railway Company must pretend that it has nothing to do with politics or the military."[9]

Upon the sudden death of Kodama, in 1906, Gotō was persuaded to accept the presidency of the South Manchuria Railway to continue the work and vision of Kodama. Gotō's approach in Manchuria was, in outline, the same as he had used in Taiwan: good relations with the local peoples, recruitment of young, highly qualified personnel, and a heavy dose of "research."

In addition to its obvious function as a railway company, the South Manchuria Railway was a central vehicle for state policy in Manchuria. The railway management there enjoyed close relations with the Japanese cabinet and with the military in Manchuria. The railways in Manchuria were seen as central to its commercial development and modernization. As part of Japanese colonial strategy, Gotō adapted the narrow Japanese railway gauge to match that of the Chinese and Korean gauge of 4 feet 8 1/2 inches rather than the Russian gauge of 5 feet. Gotō saw an integrated rail system as essential for large-scale colonization of North China. At the same time, this plan denied Russia easy access to this growing system.

The South Manchuria Railway infiltrated the towns and villages adjacent to its lines by the construction of roads, sewage systems, bridges, water supplies, hospitals, parks, and cemeteries.

World-class resort hotels were built along the railroads and staffed by European-trained hotel managers. An aggressive advertising campaign was designed to bring tourists to Manchuria and to make the South Manchuria Railway part of an international transportation system, the fastest way from Japan to Europe.[10] The South Manchuria Railway research department, with its many sections, produced mountains of reports on almost every conceivable aspect of Manchuria. Indeed, it was said that the research department was much larger than the actual railway operations. That view was in keeping with the Japanese view that the railway was primarily an instrument of colonization and only secondarily a transportation company. This concept was summed up in Gotō's favorite policy slogan: "Bunsōtelo bubi" (Military preparedness behind cultural projects).[11]

Gotō was indefatigable and was described by some critics as "a maniac in building hospitals and water systems everywhere he went."[12] Indeed, the medical and public health infrastructure in South Manchuria was impressive and was ready and adaptable when faced with the threat of plague a few years later.

In Manchuria Japan certainly had the most well developed, comprehensive, and subtle diplomacy of all the Great Powers. Not only did Japanese diplomats seem to have a better understanding of China based on long-term study and common cultural assumptions, but Japan's Manchurian policies hit closer to home than those of the other foreign powers. For Europeans and the United States, Manchuria was simply a puzzle piece in the incipient globalization that would come to characterize the twentieth century.

Whereas the thoughts of Roosevelt and the German Kaiser reflected so-called Grand Strategy, the geopolitical drama played out on smaller scales wherever and whenever the opportunity presented itself. Skirmishes over customs inspections, railway regulations, and even antiplague measures were the local stages for these events. We have an especially detailed account of one such scene in the Japanese-Chinese struggle from the small town of Antung in Manchuria. It illustrates clearly the intimate entanglement of public health needs and broader geopolitical concerns.

Antung is a town about twenty-five miles upstream from the mouth of the Yalu River, which separates Manchuria from Korea. The Korean town just opposite is Sinuiju, now connected by a major bridge over the Yalu and still one of the few ways to enter Korea by land from the north. Sinuiju (new Uiju) was founded by Japanese interests in 1910 nearer the proposed bridge site than the existing Korean town of Uiju, seven miles upstream. Antung is the terminus of one of the newly improved routes belonging to the South Manchuria Railway Company, known as the Mukden-Antung line. It served to exploit an important lumbering industry along the Yalu River. Even so, it was a city of minor importance to international commerce; the foreign diplomatic presence consisted of only two nations: Kibe Moriichi, who was the senior consul, represented Japan, and E. Carlton Baker, newly arrived in Antung in 1909, represented the United States.[13] According to diplomatic protocol, Kibe, as the senior member of Antung's diplomatic core (usually referred to as the doyen or dean), was the person who represented the collective foreign interests in negotiations with the Chinese authorities. Just across the Yalu River, Kibe's colleagues were by this time in full control. The Japan-Korea Annexation Treaty, sometimes known in Korea as the "Humiliation of the Nation in the Year of the Dog," was signed on 22 August 1910 and started the de facto Japanese rule in Korea.[14]

In January 1911, when the epidemic was spreading rapidly along the railway routes, the Chinese were particularly concerned that it might arrive in Antung at any moment via the Mukden-

Antung line. Customs authorities in Antung were eager to implement sanitary regulations to control railway traffic from Mukden,
where the plague was raging. Baker wrote to his superiors in both
Peking and Washington with a vivid description of Japanese tactics at the local level:

> The question of Sanitary Regulations for Antung has always been
> a vexing one on account of local conditions which are peculiar. The
> Japanese officials are very jealous of any power or authority exercised
> by the [Chinese] Imperial Maritime Customs because it is settled
> policy of Japan to extend her jurisdiction at Antung as far as possible
> and to ignore the rights of China. The disposition, also, of the Japa-
> nese to set up their authority in Antung is reflected in the attitude of
> the Senior Consul, who is Japanese, toward his only colleague here,
> the American Consul [Baker]. The former, instead of consulting on
> proper occasions with the latter, presumes to act independently, on
> the theory that there are at Antung only two sets of officials, the Chi-
> nese and the Japanese. . . . The Japanese Consul, also, had taken ad-
> vantage of his senior position to further the illegitimate interests of
> Japan. This, of course, has been done in a covered and indirect way
> but is deliberately planned and premeditated.[15]

Baker described the year-long attempt by the Chinese Imperial Customs Commissioner to develop Sanitary Regulations
for Antung as an international port and explained how every attempt to do so was blocked by Consul Kibe, sometimes by inaction and sometimes by petty objections. Plague, of course, was
not the only worry of the customs officials. In July 1910 there was
a cholera outbreak at Newchwang and other neighboring places
along the railroad, and Antung officials sought to develop and implement Sanitary Regulations aimed at containing that outbreak.
Kibe "stated that he had not been able to send the Sanitary Regulations to Peking [for approval], but that he would shortly do so."
But, as Baker went on to explain: "With the outbreak of cholera

. . . the local Japanese authorities in the absence of Customs Sanitary Regulations sought to examine vessels under the Japanese flag by means of the Japanese Antung Police Department. Realizing the significance of this move, I privately urged the Commissioner of Customs to take the matter of quarantine into his own hands and draw up Provisional Sanitary Regulations to cover the situation."[16]

When plague became an immediate concern in Antung in January 1911 the consular body in Peking "authorized the Chinese government to immediately enforce at Antung the same Sanitary Regulations as those already accepted by the same body for the other ports." Mr. Kibe apparently ignored this directive and, according to Consul Baker, stated to the commissioner of customs that a previous, very mild set of regulations first proposed in 1909 would be acceptable to the Japanese. These regulations applied only to traffic on the Yalu River, which at the time was frozen solid, not to the active threat posed by railway traffic from infected areas. The commissioner tried to apply very general provisions of these regulations to railway traffic, but "this suggestion on the part of Mr. Holwill was promptly rejected by Mr. Kibe who stated that the Japanese authorities could never permit such an assumption of authority on the part of Chinese officials. Mr. Holwill, however, stated that no other arrangement would be suitable and that he would endeavor to bring it about." Nonetheless, through intimidation of the Chinese officials and further inaction, Kibe managed to scuttle any attempts to implement Sanitary Regulations at Antung. On 18 January Holwill sent Kibe an "ultimatum" with respect to implementation of the updated Sanitary Regulations from Peking, and again, on 19 January, Kibe stonewalled: "I am not in a position to consent to the proposed notification being given which is based on a reading of the said Regulations contrary to our views." As Baker analyzed this exchange: "I have no doubt, however, that the thought of jurisdiction and the exercise of sovereign rights is uppermost in his mind, though he will not likely discuss the political features of the situation except as a last resort."[17]

As Baker explained to Washington,

> It is obvious, of course, that the real issue at stake is not so much with Sanitary Regulations as with the broader question of Japanese jurisdiction in Manchuria. The Japanese no doubt would rather see one hundred or even a thousand persons die of the plague in Antung that to give up any part of the jurisdiction which they now assume. If they can resist successfully the exercise of Customs authority over goods coming from the North by railway, they could likely follow the same course with respect to persons and goods coming by rail from Korea after the completion of the new Yalu River Bridge.[18]

Baker, an astute political observer, noted a subtle Japanese tactic in China. Given the power of the foreign diplomatic presence, deriving in the main from the management of the Boxer indemnities, the Japanese were quietly maintaining their consuls in Chinese locations for long periods so that by 1911, as Baker noted, "the Japanese have Senior Consuls in nearly every port in Manchuria and . . . the American Government has failed to place at these cities Consuls who would be likely to make a thorough study of Chinese affairs and to remain at the same place for a reasonable number of years [becoming the senior consul was based on time of local tenure]. It has, I believe, been partly due to this unnoticed policy that the Japanese have been able to take advantage of the Chinese in the way that they have."[19] Baker's subsequent career certainly exemplified the peripatetic existence of American diplomatic personnel.

At least from the time of the Meiji Restoration, Japan's designs on Korea and Manchuria were manifest. The outcomes of the Sino-Japanese War in 1895 and of the Russo-Japanese War in 1905 left Japan with a strong presence in South Manchuria, a presence that would eventually lead to full occupation and evolution of the puppet state of Manchukuo in 1932. The pneumonic plague in 1910–1911 provided a focus for Japan's colonial activities in South Manchuria during this critical period. It required public health and administrative cooperation with other foreign powers with interests in China, as well as with the Chinese themselves. This requirement may have tempered and, for a time, slowed the inevitable Japanese ambitions in Manchuria.

RUSSIA IN MANCHURIA

In spite of several treaties, agreements, and "secret protocols," Russia continued to be wary of Japanese intentions in Manchuria. St. Petersburg believed that Japan was "systematically making speedy preparations for a new war and was using all of South Manchuria and Korea, with their railway lines, military arsenals, and camps as a hinterland from which to attack."[20] The Russian historian Boris A. Romanov opined that "by the spring of 1909 a situation had been created which would admit of Japan's appearing in the Amur province with eleven divisions within two weeks of the opening of hostilities against Russia, after first taking a few days to liquidate Vladivostok, which was absolutely unfitted for defense by land, let alone by sea."[21]

After the Russo-Japanese War, there developed a fairly clear understanding between Japan and Russia with respect to the "spheres of influence" appropriate for each power. Japan took over Russia's rail lines and cities in the South, while Russia continued to develop and expand its development and colonial activities in the North.

The central question for Russia in the aftermath of its loss to Japan in 1905 was the proper policy with respect to hegemony in North Manchuria. While the Russian hopes for a "Yellow Russia," in the words of the scholar Rosemary Quested, were aborted by the events of 1905, Russian commercial interests and colonization were rapidly increasing, and St. Petersburg was showing interest in bringing Manchurian territories under permanent Russian control. Harbin became the focus of Russian political intrigue aimed at establishing this control. Since the Chinese Eastern Railway was under Russian control by treaty rights with China, the railway administration was central to these political efforts. The city of Harbin became the center of Russian influence in Manchuria, and until well after the Bolshevik Revolution in 1917, it was a center of Russian conservatism. Harbin was nominally a Chinese city, but its administration was in the hands of the Russians, a mix of railway officials and military officers stationed there under the guise of providing protection for the Chinese Eastern Railway administered lands.

Tax policy, tariff rules, police practices, and public health activities were all assumed by the local Russian administration of Harbin. The diplomatic records of the time document seemingly endless small disputes as the Russians sought to extend their control; meanwhile the Chinese and the local representatives of other foreign governments resisted such efforts as best they could.

From 1902 the railway administration in Harbin was under the control of General Dimitri Leonidovic Horvath, a protégé of the powerful Sergei Witte. Both Horvath and Witte were moderates who approached the Chinese with a modicum of respect and deference. General Horvath was generally viewed as a competent administrator in a difficult situation. The Russian government was divided in its attitude toward its Far East involvement, and the railway administration, entangled as it was in both economic and political realities, was notoriously fractious and inefficient. When Witte's star fell in St. Petersburg in 1906, having been forced to resign as the first imperial prime minister, Horvath's position was even more tenuous. In the fall of 1910, just as our epidemic was beginning, Alexander Izvolsky, the Russian foreign minister with reformist tendencies was replaced by Sergi Sazonov of similar sympathies. Sazonov would prove, however, more accommodating to the Japanese interests, eventually signing several treaties and secret protocols relating to mutual spheres of influence in Mongolia.

By the fall of 1910, the Chinese Eastern Railway had become a financial burden. Inept management had turned what should have been a going concern into a money-losing enterprise. Although it might have been possible to sell the Chinese Eastern Railway either to China or to an international consortium, this rail line was key to Russian domination in North Manchuria under the pretense of the railway treaties with China. Further, both the Japanese and the Russians viewed an effort by American bankers to get involved in the purchase of the Chinese Eastern Railway as a threat by the United States to establish a competing "sphere of influence" in Manchuria.[22] Without the railway operation, Russia's pretext for nearly de facto occupation of North Manchuria would be untenable. The other alternative was outright annexation of North Manchuria. This possibility came to a head at an extraordinary meeting of the Council of Ministers of Russia in St. Petersburg between 19 November and 2 December 1910, where "the Minister of Foreign Affairs declared that he was perfectly convinced that the annexation [to Russia] of Northern Manchuria was for us an imperative necessity, but, owing to the probable opposition of America and England, was at the moment inopportune. A decision was finally reached to postpone the annexation and instead to bring pressure to bear on China in protection of Russia's 'stipulated privileges' in North Manchuria, but, in case of necessity however there must be no shrinking from forceful measures."[23] This pressure soon took the form of an ultimatum to China in March 1911, in which Russia threatened China with occupation of Yining (Ghulja/Kuldja), a major city in western Xinjiang province, near the Kazakhstan border. But, in the poetic imagery of Edward Zabriskie, "the Chinese bamboo bent before the Russian wind. Peking yielded so completely on the points in question that St. Petersburg had slight ground left upon which to continue its campaign of pressure."[24] Thus, Russian hopes for their future in the Far East lingered on. Following the fall of the Qing dynasty in 1912, Sazonov, in addressing the "Mongolian Question" and recognition of the new government of Yüan Shih K'ai, noted: "The definite settlement of this difficult question [the existence of Mongolia as an autonomous component of the Chinese realm], which especially affects Russian interests, must be postponed to a future date, for we have to take into account our political interests which, in principle, are directly opposed to the maintenance of China's territorial integrity."[25]

In short, then, Russia's foothold in Manchuria continually weakened, starting with its defeat in the Russo-Japanese War and the loss of momentum of its Far East strategy. By the time of the Great Plague, its main surrogate in Manchuria, the Chinese Eastern Railway, was in financial trouble and its influence was limited to the region surrounding the railway town of Harbin. It used the occasion of the plague to exercise administrative and medical authority is ways that might bolster its local control and maintain precedents for its hegemony in North Manchuria. In contrast to earlier times, however, the other Western powers, together with the Chinese, were able to effectively blunt many of these attempts. The days of a Russian Manchuria were clearly numbered.

CHINA IN MANCHURIA

As the plague spread southward in Manchuria, China faced other serious challenges in the south. Long-smoldering political unrest led by a tenuous coalition of warlords, anti-Qing reformers, and populist revolutionaries spawned the Wuchang uprising in 1910 and demands for a national parliament and more popular government. By the winter of 1910 it was becoming clear that events were outpacing the capacity of the central Chinese government to deal with them. The increasing decentralized rule in which provincial governors, and in the case of Manchuria, the viceroy, had more and more independence worked well enough to deal with regional problems such as local management of the plague, but for national and international challenges, the imperial court was too weak to fend off its foes. Relentless pressures from Russia and, especially, Japan proved constant worries. The rise of Han nationalism and anti-Manchu racism further complicated Qing politics.[26] The dramatic rise in population in Manchuria due to Han immigration only exacerbated these tensions.[27]

As argued by Pamela Crossley, the decline of the Qing dynasty certainly began with the rise of the Taiping rebellion in southern China, a product of social unrest and anti-Manchu sentiment that resulted in one of the deadliest civil wars in history, from 1850 to 1864, along with another uprising in the north of China called the Nian rebellion.[28] Although the Qing dynasty managed to suppress these challenges, it was weakened in many ways that led, ultimately, to its demise following the October 1911 uprisings in central China and the establishment of the Republic of China.

While the stage was being set for the explosion of the plague, the Qing government was struggling with attempts at modernization in Manchuria. A transition from the Banner System to privatization, the so-called new policy, was implemented from 1902 to 1912 in attempts to counter the "debt and threat" from both within and without. It was more interventionist and established a "land reclamation bureau" to seize and sell land to Han Chinese to block Russian advances.[29] In April 1907 an imperial decree abolished the Tartar generalship and appointed a viceroy who was also the imperial high commissioner, thus providing the authority to command imperial troops from outside his own region. The viceroy was henceforth able to rule and administer on the same basis as the governors of the other eighteen provinces. Governors, who also held the title of major-general, with command authority over Manchus and Mongols in their provinces, were appointed for each of the three provinces. The Japanese region, that is, the Leased Territories, had a military governor-general under the direction of the minister of foreign affairs of Japan, who controlled the civil and military administration, the courts, and the South Manchuria Railway in his domain.[30]

MEDICINE BETWEEN COLONIAL
AND POSTCOLONIAL TIMES

Historical discourse on the development of non-Western countries is overwhelmingly framed in terms of colonialism and its aftermath. This is especially true in the case of medicine and public health. The role and conception of health and sickness have been invoked as central to both modernization and nationhood.

Mark Harrison, in his sweeping account of disease and the modern world, asserts, "I aim to show that disease was central to the development of modern states and their machinery of government."[31] Other scholars, too, have emphasized the importance of medicine and public health in the colonial enterprise, as well as a means to understand history more generally. Zinsser and McNeill put disease front and center as an important historical cause (an "actor," in modern jargon).[32] Yet in the case of China, and Manchuria in particular, this framework is more complex. China, while subject to repeated assaults from the Great Powers, including Japan, was not truly colonized, and except for some specific instances was at least nominally sovereign over its territory.

The responses to the plague in Manchuria represented not so much an evolution of colonial practices or a postcolonial hybrid of one sort or another, but rather a varied mixture of colonial policies, local practices, and ad hoc efforts. Coming at a time when the failing Qing government was faced with rebellion in the south and in Shanghai, challenges on the international stage, and traditionally weak central control of the provinces, the emergency of the plague in Manchuria seemed to result in an abrogation of responsibility, leaving it to the various local groups that might rise to the occasion. As Judith Farquhar has noted: "Wherever medical work has emerged as a genre of practice, it is often messy and smelly and most of the time very mundane."[33] Such a statement could well characterize the hodgepodge efforts to deal with the great Manchurian plague.

The Manchurian context varied from place to place depending on the local mix of foreign and Chinese influence. In Russian Harbin, the quasi-military approach to quarantine was dominant. In Japanese Dairen, the softer, yet just as insistent, velvet glove diplomacy of the public health expert Gotō Shinpei was tempered by the harder military authority of the Kwantung Army. In between, in Mukden, we see a more Chinese approach, yet undoubtedly Western in its motivation. As Ruth Rogaski has argued, public health in China was imbued with the entire project of modernization and the agenda of the late Qing reformers. She traces the concept and term *weisheng* from its traditional meaning of self-cultivation to a much broader concept of sovereignty, identity, and responsibility for the national welfare, captured in her term "hygienic modernity."[34] As several observers have suggested, the legacy of the responses to the Manchurian plague would shape the development of both the notion of public health as well as the recognition of Western medicine as state medicine in China.[35]

In contrast to the interplay of the colonial power with the subsequent postcolonial government as Anderson has described in the Philippines, where the American public health model was adopted and then adapted by the Filipinos, in China, a more eclectic development occurred.[36] To be sure, it was infused with Western concepts and practices, but as Rogaski has suggested, the mediating role of the Japanese as an already Westernized yet Asian nation made such transitions more immediately acceptable.[37] The rhetoric of postcolonial studies often employs the concepts of resistance and acceptance, yet again these notions may not apply so simply to Manchuria.[38] In Harbin, major resistance seems to have come not from the local Chinese and Korean inhabitants but from the non-Russian Westerners, the businessmen and foreign diplomatic community, fearful of precedents set by the Russian administrators that under other circumstances would have been viewed as reasonable, but instead were seen as preludes to even tighter Russian hegemony.

The Japanese preparedness in the Leased Territories of the

southern Liaotung peninsula was both massive and, probably, effective in channeling the plague to the southwest and away from Dairen. The resistance of the Chinese in the Leased Territories seems to be minimal, probably the result of the careful colonizing policies of Japan, aimed at ingratiating the Japanese rule over the local population. These policies were, of course, followed repeatedly as Japan styled itself as the "white Asian" nation in its vision as the leader of a Greater East Asia Co-Prosperity Sphere.

The post-Qing development of Westernized institutions aimed at epidemic diseases in North China, in particular plague and cholera, would contribute to the ongoing changes in both medicine and public health. The prestige accorded China on the international front from having handled the challenges of the Manchurian plague and the postplague conference in Mukden would further its "hygienic modernity" as well as its self-confidence as a nation capable of modern science. The embrace of scientism and of "Mr. Science" as a national icon in the 1920s was certainly helped by this early success.[39]

By the summer of 1911 the plague was past, the Qing dynasty was no more, and Russian ambitions in Manchuria were becoming increasingly unrealistic. But Manchuria was still a land in turmoil. As a Chinese borderland, it was still not fully integrated into Chinese national consciousness, not secure from foreign designs, and not able to chart its own course with confidence. The Great Plague had been a challenge, a disruption, and one of those unforeseen contingencies that constrain and channel the course of human events. For China, it was one of many stresses that contributed to the rapidity of the final days of the Qing; for its neighbors, it was an opportunity to be exploited as best they could for their own geopolitical goals. A succinct and fitting summary of the situation was provided by the United States minister in Peking, William J. Calhoun, to Secretary of State Philander Knox: [40]

> To sum up the foregoing: the situation in Manchuria was serious. Both Russia and Japan had large vested interests in the country, and a large number of their nationals were residents therein. These powers might well claim that, if any outside influence interfered, they should have the first right to do so, because they had the largest interest to protect; and, according to Doctor Kitazato [*sic*], Japan, at least was best qualified to cope with the situation. Therefore, both Russia and Japan might well be expected to object to the introduction of any international body, however disinterested its motive. Any suggestion of that kind could well be construed as an admission that the Chinese had failed, that the necessities of the situation required or justified outside interference; and the only effect would be to stimulate both Japan and Russia to step in and take control of Manchuria, and to retain such control for all time.

> This was the situation, and the foregoing were the reasons which made me doubt the expediency of even suggesting the introduction of an international body of any kind. If the Japanese had moved another division of troops and taken charge, who, as the German Chargé d'Affaires said to me the other day, would there have been to object but the Chinese, and what would they have done? Nothing. Happily the plague has passed away; the danger for the time being is averted; but the shadow of threatening possibilities still hangs low and heavy over ill fated Manchuria.[41]

A Century Later

Since 1910, medical knowledge of plague and other epidemic infectious diseases has grown to an unimagined and, indeed, nearly unmanageable extent. Yet, just as surprising, in several ways very little has changed. The twenty-first-century plague fighter has an impressive array of antibiotics to deploy, rapid laboratory tests to use, and global communication networks to access. Just the same, recent epidemics have been fraught with many of the challenges of the great Manchurian plague of 1910–1911.

To highlight these parallels, one need only consider a few widespread epidemic diseases of the intervening century: influenza, plague, Nipah virus, severe acute respiratory syndrome (SARS), and HIV. Flu and HIV seem to have progressed from epidemic threats to fluctuating endemic infections. Plague outbreaks are rare but significant, and SARS and Nipah, thus far at least, seem to have been essentially singular occurrences. In addition, the ancient global scourges of malaria and tuberculosis remain well entrenched.

Influenza is rivaled only by HIV as the most lethal epidemic disease of the past century, but the others offer interesting comparisons as well. All these epidemics, like the Manchurian plague, have their origins in the ecology of human-nonhuman interactions. Flu is primarily an infection of birds, yet it can frequently adapt to become pathogenic and highly transmissible among both pigs and humans.[1] Nipah, perhaps less well known, appears to be a virus carried by bats in Southeast and South Asia that can be quite lethal to humans when transmitted via pigs. Recent outbreaks of Nipah have been blamed on habitat degradation that brings domestic pigs into closer contact with jungle-dwelling bats.[2] Likewise, HIV is a virus that originated, at least prior to its human phase, in wild African monkeys.[3] All these examples illustrate an essentially ecological viewpoint that emerged in the study of the Manchurian plague.

Ecology of disease involves several levels of analysis: the cellular, the organismal, and the populational. Consider disease at the cellular level: the causative organism, for example, the plague bacillus or the influenza virus, interacts with the cells of its hosts in specific ways, depending on virus receptor structure, toxin binding sites, or routes of inoculation. Some diseases are highly species-specific, while others are more promiscuous pathogens. Smallpox virus and poliovirus, for example, naturally infect only humans. Cholera bacteria produce a toxin that affects only the cells of the gastrointestinal tract of humans. Other diseases, such as influenza, have much wider host ranges. Plague bacilli infect both rodents and humans and, in addition, are carried in a viable form by insects. As scientific knowledge increased during the twentieth century, the reasons for such natural susceptibility and resistance to infectious diseases gradually became known. We now understand why farmers catch flu but not hog cholera from their pigs, and why humans never get canine distemper.

This understanding of the biology of host-parasite interactions, or the cellular ecology of infectious diseases, provides the basis for another level of disease ecology, that based on the whole organism and its interactions. The obligatory role of two distinct organisms in some diseases is now clear. So-called intermediate hosts are organisms that are intermediary in the passage of the disease agent from one species to another. Well-known examples include malaria, which requires mosquitoes both for part of the life cycle of the parasite as well as for efficient spread from human to human, and schistosomiasis, for which aquatic snails provide an intermediate host for part of the parasite's life cycle. Adaptation and mutation of both host and parasite can lead to changes in the disease spectrum over time. Sometimes this ecological concept involves the notion of "jumping the species barrier," so that a previously unknown animal disease becomes pathogenic for humans. Ever since humans domesticated animals, and probably for even earlier hunter-gatherer cultures, zoonoses, or diseases that infect animals, have been important to humans as well. We are close to our animals—so close, in fact, that we share diseases.

Disease ecology also involves social and functional interactions between species. Until biologists began to take ecology seriously in the 1930s, however, the close relationship between human and animal health was not fully appreciated. Although there were specific examples such as milk-borne tuberculosis and undulant fever, saliva-borne rabies, and animal anthrax as the source of wool-sorters disease, animals as a natural reservoir of disease that could trouble human beings were largely ignored. As we experience cultural changes in what we eat, the animals we interact with, and the animal products we use, human beings encounter animal pathogens in new and varied ways. In the past we viewed our diseases from our usual anthropocentric vantage, assuming that they were, indeed, *our* diseases. Only lately have we come to realize that frequently we are only the occasional victim of a predominantly animal infection. One reason for this hubris, of course, is that infections can be inapparent or subclinical, with no obvious symptoms in some host species. Thus, asymptomatic carrier states mask infection. Flu in wild ducks may not be obvious, but when the ducks transmit the virus to domestic swine, and hence to humans, it is easier to recognize the proximate source, that is, the poor pig, rather than the true natural reservoir of influenza epidemics.

The plague in Manchuria illuminates three conceptual levels: the cultural and social, the ecological, and the biomedical. In the case of this pneumonic plague, the role of the Siberian marmot and its ecological relationship to human hunting practices and culture were essential features in the understanding and control of this epidemic. This appreciation of the subtle connections between microbe, marmot, and humans was a first in epidemiological history. In no previous pestilence was such a nuanced understanding possible. Of course the association of rats and plague had been noted since at least the fourteenth century, but without seeing the disease as a natural unfolding of biological interrelationships. In the intervening hundred years since the Manchurian plague, epidemiologists have come to think of such ecological relationships as fundamental to their discipline: disease ecology, community health, biological equilibria, host-parasite interactions, herd immunity, and natural reservoirs of disease have all become common concepts.[4] Without these notions, which were elaborated in embryonic form during the great Manchurian plague, insect-borne diseases such as yellow fever, malaria, and more recently Lyme disease and West Nile fever would be much harder to understand and control. Without recognition of the importance of animal reservoirs (or lack of such reservoirs), the successful smallpox eradication campaign of the 1960s and 1970s would not have been attempted. Monitoring of both wild and domestic avian species for influenza virus strains provides important advance warning of potential human epidemics on a global scale.[5]

Population and social ecology provide another, even more complex story. On the diplomatic front, too, the Manchurian plague presaged twentieth-century approaches to other epidemics. The great cholera epidemics of the nineteenth century were recognized as global problems, and by midcentury international cooperation and consensus were being mobilized to combat them, for example, by the International Sanitary Conferences, first held in Paris in 1851. It was not until the end of 1907, however, that the Office International d'Hygiène Publique (OIHP) was established in Paris with the broader aim to consider issues beyond cholera; later the epidemiological role of OIHP evolved into part of the World Health Organization (WHO) under the United Nations. The ten International Sanitary Conferences in the nineteenth century were all held in response to the perceived invasion of Europe by cholera from Asia, and the seven Sanitary Conferences between 1874 and 1897 were devoted to the diplomatic and political attempts to control cholera by quarantines and interdictions. A key target of these efforts was the great migration associated with the annual Muslim pilgrimage to Mecca, the hadj, with its associated cholera outbreaks, and a key point of control was Suez, where a sanitary station was established under international control to act as a barrier to "Asian" diseases entering Europe.[6]

To this day, the conflicts between the transnational demands of public health and the protection of national sovereignty confound all global responses to epidemic disease. Sometimes international cooperation has been improbably effective: during the height of the Cold War, the United States and the Soviet Union cooperated in the successful global eradication of smallpox. Sometimes such cooperation has been amazingly sluggish, if not downright obstructive, as in the puzzling Chinese response to the SARS epidemic in early 2003, when sick patients were removed from hospitals and driven around Beijing in vans and ambulances to hide them from visiting WHO epidemiologists.[7]

In the devastating influenza pandemic of 1918, the exigencies of World War I influenced public health policy in the United States and abroad.[8] Again, secrecy prevailed and effective measures were delayed, if not entirely suppressed. President Wilson's focus on total war and maintaining morale at all costs led to influenza deaths on a massive scale. Against the counsel of his own medical advisers, Wilson sent thousands of American troops to die of the "Spanish" flu aboard transport ships en route to Europe in support of the United States' cause there. Again, the intersection of political demands, disease ecology, and medical knowledge was manifest in these casualties. With hindsight, all is clear; at the time, perhaps it was not. As in the case of the Manchurian plague, knowledge of epidemic disease was fragmentary. Organisms, their modes of transmission, their diagnosis, the roles of carriers, and effective treatments, both curative and supportive, were usually not appreciated or even known by the most expert medical scientists. In the face of expert uncertainty, political pressures are hard to resist.

By mid-twentieth century, in the postwar glow of international cooperation before the onset of the virulent East-West Cold War competition, the United Nations gave birth to a global health organization of rather remarkable effectiveness and resiliency, the World Health Organization. What is remarkable about the WHO is not its failures and successes so much as its existence as an effective agency at all. The WHO has managed to exist for more than sixty years as an organization that finds ways to blunt national political interests, cajole international cooperation to face global health problems, and maintain widespread scientific credibility. In 1910 the Manchurian plague was seen as a global threat, and was met by the piecemeal actions of Japan, Russia, and China, each with its own geopolitical ax to grind. One hundred years later, such national self-interests are tempered by the WHO as an outside body of expertise and advice to curb local and regional proclivities aimed at parochial advantage. Like the International Plague Conference in Mukden in April 1911, the WHO gets its effectiveness and credibility from the scientists and physicians who form part of what some have called "the invisible college," transnational communities of experts who share common beliefs about science and medical practice, who have collaborated on research projects in the past, who have shared teachers and mentors, and who see their calling as essentially apolitical.[9] Some scholars have made distinctions between overtly political and diplomatic organizations, on one hand, and agencies like the WHO that, while subject to political pressures, have functional roles based on technical expertise that are not primarily political and are aimed at generally agreed-upon humanitarian goals. Such international networks of scientists, from Mukden in 1911 to Geneva in the twenty-first century, serve as a counterweight to the nationally focused work of diplomats and politicians.

One aspect of epidemic disease that is often overlooked as well as potentially paradoxical is its role in advancing scientific and medical knowledge. To borrow from Willie Sutton, "One studies epidemics because that is where the diseases are." During major epidemics, scientists have often been able to achieve an understanding of a disease that would have been impossible under normal conditions. When the bubonic plague struck Hong Kong in 1895, no living physician had experienced a major plague epidemic, and the only available knowledge was from classical texts such as Sydenham's account of the London plague of 1665, over two centuries earlier. The autopsies, the bacteriological examinations, and the epidemiological data from the Manchurian plague provided a valuable mass of information on pneumonic plague that had never before been collected. To this day, the publications of Wu Lien-Teh and Robert Pollitzer based on this and subsequent outbreaks in Manchuria are still authoritative.[10] From influenza to polio to SARS, it has been during periods of epidemic flare-ups that medical science has had the research material, in terms of patients, populations, and public support, to make major advances in understanding these diseases.

What differences can we observe between the geopolitical responses to disease at the beginning of the twentieth century and those of the twenty-first? For one thing, responses have become more formal, more well organized, and more predictable, representing entrenched organizational structures. In 1911 the Office International d'Hygiène Publique was only four years old and was the only truly international body devoted to international health. A century later there are both intergovernmental organizations with huge staffing, large budgets, and global reach as well as myriad large and small nongovernmental organizations devoted to both local and transnational health issues. Some of these bodies are clearly agents of national and regional politics, such as the Pan American Health Organization. The World Health Assembly, the forum through which the WHO is governed, is often hampered by the intrusion of geopolitical rivalries to the detriment of its global health mission.

The recognition of the economic consequences of epidemics,

of course, can be seen at least as early as the great plagues of the early modern period. The Black Death in Florence was described by Boccaccio and others as devastating to the normal commerce of the city.[11] Defoe's fictional account the London plague of 1665 was told through the diary of a small merchant who wrote of its effects on his business.[12] As we have seen, in the Manchurian plague, too, the economic impact was central to the responses mounted by all the actors involved.

What is particularly interesting now, early in the twenty-first century, is the key role assumed by the World Bank in funding, directing, and promoting public health activities around the globe. Whereas in China during the early twentieth century, economic interests such as those of international bankers seeking to bankroll Chinese railroads were the background to the geopolitics in Manchuria, by the early twenty-first century, economic justifications of public health efforts, for example, for antimalaria campaigns in Africa and clean water programs worldwide, have taken stage front and center.[13] More than humanitarian concerns, economic justifications now seem to drive responses to global epidemics. The close connection between economic health and physical health is now an unquestioned assumption of policy makers and development experts. A healthy workforce is now seen as a key requirement for economic prosperity.

Another difference is the well-established view that ecological approaches are central to global epidemiology. The integration of environmental science and epidemiology is one of the major conceptual advances of the past century. This broadened view has been applied to twentieth-century concerns such as insect vector control in the cases of malaria eradication, yellow fever campaigns, Dutch elm disease, food inspections in the case of the spongiform encephalopathies (for example, mad cow disease), and alerts about global warming in the case of expanding habitats of disease vectors, to mention just a few well-established examples.

In retrospect, we see little unique about the Manchurian plague except that it occurred at a time when new knowledge of microbes was just awaiting epidemiological application, and it occurred at a place of sufficient importance to world powers that major resources and attention were focused there. It was a fortuitous quirk of history that individuals of talent, experience, and dedication became involved. Such a conjunction of the right knowledge, the right resources, and the right people has not always been the case in other global challenges of epidemic disease.

Appendix
Place Names in Manchuria

Contemporary Name	Current Name (Province)	Other Forms
Aigun	Aihui (Heilongjiang)	Aihun, Ta hei ho
Amur River	Heilongjiang	Heilungjiang, Heilungkiang
Antung	Dandong (Liaoning)	Andong, Ngantung
Beichan	Beicheng (Jilin)	
Ch'ang ch'un	Changchun (Jilin)	
Ch'ing tao	Qingdao (Shandong)	Tsingtao
Chou t'sun	Unidentified rail station in Jilin	
Daiboshin	Dalianwanzhen (Liaoning)	Ta Fang Shen
Dairen	Dalian (Liaoning)	Dalny/Dal'ni, Talien
Feng t'ien	Shenyang (Liaoning)	Fung t'ien, Mukden
Fuchiatien	Harbin (Heilongjiang)	
Fushan	Fushan coal field (Liaoning)	
Hailar	Hailar (Heilongjiang)	Hulun, Khailar
Hailun	Hailun (Heilongjiang)	
Harbin	Harbin (Heilongjiang)	Haer bin, Ha erh pin
Irkutsk	Irkutsk (Irkutsk Oblast, Russia)	

Contemporary Name	Current Name (Province)	Other Forms
Kaichou	Gaizhou (Liaoning)	Kaiping
Kiaochow	Jiaozhou (Shandong)	Kiautschou
Kirin	Jilin City (Jilin)	Kilin
Kuan ch'eng tze	Section of Changchun (Jilin)	
Kwantung	Parts of Liaoning and Jilin	Leased Territories
Lahasusu	Tongjiang (Heilongjiang)	Tungchiang
Liaotung	Liaodong peninsula (Liaoning)	
Manchouli	Manzhouli (Inner Mongolia)	Manchuria Station
Mukden	Shenyang (Liaoning)	Shengjing, Fengtian
Nanshan	Jinzhou (Liaoning)	Kinchou, Chin chou
Nerchinsk	Nerchinsk (Russia)	Nibuchu
Newchwang	Yingkou (Liaoning)	Niuzhuang, Niuchwang, Ying Kow, Inkow
Pechili	Bohai (Gulf of)	
Peiyang University	Tianjin University	
Peking	Beijing	Peiping
Port Arthur	Lüshun (Liaoning)	
Shanhaikuan	Shanhaiguan (Hebei)	Shanhaikwan
Shantung	Shandong	
Sungari River	Songhuajiang	
Tashihchiao	Dashiqiao (Liaoning)	Da Chi Zhao
Tientsin	Tianjin	
Tsitsihar	Qiqihar (Heilongjiang)	Tsitsikar, Tsitsicar
Tungchou	Tongzhou (Beijing)	Tongxian, Tungshow
Transbaikalia	Amur Oblast, Russia Buryat Republic, and Zabaykalsky Krai of Russian Federation	
Yentai	Yentai coal field (Liaoning)	
Yining	Gulja (Xinjiang)	Ghulja, Kuldja

Notes

CHAPTER 1: PLAGUE COMES TO MANCHURIA

1. Correspondent in China, "Notes from China," *Lancet* 1 (1911): 775.

2. Manchuria is a problematic designation for the northeastern part of present-day China. Its use in this work does not signify a recognition of this part of China as a separate entity either as proposed by the imperial Japanese government in the 1920s and 1930s (Manchukuo) or otherwise. This designation is used in its historical sense because it was the designation most often used in the sources at the time covered by this book. As Lattimore noted, "It [the name Manchuria] derives from the fact that foreign rivalry for control of China in the later nineteenth century first made Manchuria a region to be dealt with as a whole." Prior to that, the southern, agricultural region was quite sinicized, while the northern, forested, and steppe regions were distinctly separate. See Owen Lattimore, *Inner Asian Frontiers of China* (Boston: Beacon, 1962), 103–109.

3. Joseph P. Byrne, ed., *Encyclopedia of Pestilence, Pandemics, and Plagues* (Westport, Conn.: Greenwood, 2008), *s.v.* "Plague of Justinian."

4. Robert Pollitzer, *Plague* (Geneva: World Health Organization, 1954); Joseph P. Byrne, *Daily Life During the Black Death* (Westport, Conn.: Greenwood, 2006).

5. Carol Benedict, *Bubonic Plague in Nineteenth-Century China* (Stanford: Stanford University Press, 1996).

6. Guy de Chauliac, *Inventarium sive chirurgia magna* (1363), ed. Michael R. McVaugh (Leiden: E. J. Brill, 1997).

7. Ann G. Carmichael, *Plague and the Poor in Renaissance Florence* (Cambridge: Cambridge University Press, 1986), 10.

8. "Human Plague—India," *Morbidity and Mortality Weekly Report* 43 (1994): 689-691.

9. Shi Daonan, 1765-1792, in Benedict, *Bubonic Plague*, 23.

10. Alexandre Émile Jean Yersin, "La peste bubonique à Hong Kong," *Ann. Inst. Pasteur* 8 (1894): 662-667. Also see Yersin, "La peste bubonique à Hong Kong," *Comptes rendus de l'Académie des sciences* 119 (1894): 356, and Shibasaburo Kitasato, "The Bacillus of Bubonic Plague," *Lancet* 2 (1894): 428.

11. David J. Bibel and T. H. Chen, "Diagnosis of Plaque: An Analysis of the Yersin-Kitasato Controversy," *Bacteriological Reviews* 40 (1976): 633-651.

12. Tohiu Ishigami (rev. by Shibasaburo Kitasato), *Japanese Text-Book on Plague* (Adelaide: Vardon and Pritchard, 1905), 6-8.

13. See, e.g., Mark Harrison, *Disease in the Modern World* (Cambridge: Polity, 2004), 129-130; the eminent experts Burnet and White credit only Kitasato, while the equally authoritative experts Dubos and Hirsch correctly credit only Yersin; MacFarland Burnet and David O. White, *Natural History of Infectious Disease*, 4th ed. (Cambridge: Cambridge University Press, 1972), 228; René J. Dubos and James G. Hirsch, *Bacterial and Mycotic Infections of Man*, 4th ed. (Philadelphia: J. B. Lippincott, 1965), 664.

14. Paul-Louis Simond, "La propagation de la peste," *Ann. Inst. Pasteur* 12 (1898): 625-687.

15. Contagionism is a concept dating from at least the fourteenth century based on the belief that a disease can be acquired by contact or exposure to an agent or influence. It implies an external "cause." The specific agent or influence is not crucial to belief in the general theory of contagionism. Infection, on the other hand, is a more recent (nineteenth-century) conceptual refinement based on one or another germ theory of disease.

16. Masanori Ogata, "Ueber die Pestepidemie in Formosa," *Zentralblatt Bakt.* Abt. 1, 21 (1897): 769-777.

17. "A Case of Plague," *North-China Herald* (Shanghai), 28 October 1910, 231.

18. Ivan L. Martinevskii and Henri H. Mollaret, *Epidemiia chumy v Man'chzhurii v 1910–1911 gg.* (Epidemic plague in Manchuria in 1910–1911) (Moscow: Medicina, 1971).

19. Ibid., 16.

20. Ibid.

21. Ibid., 17.

22. Frank G. Clemow, "Plague in Siberia and Mongolia and the Tarbagan (*Arcomys bobac*)," *Journal of Tropical Medicine* 3 (1900): 169–174.

23. Martinevskii and Mollaret, *Epidemiia*, 24.

24. Rosemary K. I. Quested, *"Matey" Imperialists?: The Tsarist Russians in Manchuria, 1895–1917* (Hong Kong: University of Hong Kong, 1982), 105. Quested also reports that Russians and Chinese were treated together. Physician shortages in the more remote areas were also noted.

25. Wu Lien-Teh, *Plague Fighter: The Autobiography of a Modern Chinese Physician* (Cambridge: Hefter, 1959).

26. Carl F. Nathan, *Plague Prevention and Politics in Manchuria, 1910–1911* (Cambridge: Harvard East Asian Monographs, 1967).

27. Mark Gamsa, "The Epidemic of Pneumonic Plague in Manchuria, 1910–1911," *Past and Present* 190 (2006): 147–183.

28. Joseph H. Cha, "Epidemics in China," in William H. McNeill, *Plagues and Peoples* (Oxford: Blackwell, 1976), 293–302.

29. Benedict, *Bubonic Plague*, 2.

30. See Benedict, *Bubonic Plague*, and Myron Eschenberg, *Plague Ports: The Global Impact of Bubonic Plague, 1894–1901* (New York: New York University Press, 2007).

31. Marilyn Chase, *The Barbary Plague: The Black Death in Victorian San Francisco* (New York: Random House, 2003).

32. Giovanna Morelli et al., *"Yersinia pestis* Genome Sequencing Identifies Patterns of Global Phylogenetic Diversity," *Nature Genetics* 42 (2010): 1140–1143.

33. See Gamsa, "The Epidemic"; Martinevskii and Mollaret, *Epidemiia*; and Wu, *Plague Fighter.*

34. British Delegate to the Constantinople Board of Health, "Recent Plague Outbreaks in Russia and the Far East," *Lancet* 1 (1911): 59.

35. Correspondent, *North-China Herald* (Shanghai), 23 December 1910, 705.

36. *North-China Herald* (Shanghai), 20 January 1911, 157.

37. Ibid., 125.

38. Reginald Farrar, "Plague in Manchuria," *Proceedings of the Royal Society of Medicine* 5, pt. 2 (1912): 6.

39. Ibid., 3.

40. The number of tarbagan pelts exported from Manchuria by four Russian companies alone was reported at over 2 million annually; "International Plague Conference at Mukden," *Lancet* 1 (1911): 1383.

41. See Sumiko Otsubo, "The Female Body and Eugenic Thought in Meiji Japan," in *Building a Modern Japan: Science, Technology, and Medicine in the Meiji Era and Beyond*, ed. Morris Low (New York: Palgrave, 2005), 63–64. See also Morris Low, "The Japanese Nation in Evolution: W. E. Griffis, Hybridity and Whiteness of the Japanese Race," *History and Anthropology* 11 (1999): 203–234.

42. It was later generally agreed by microbiologists, historians, and even Kitasato himself that the organism described by Kitasato was not the causative agent in plague, but rather a common contaminant. The honors for the discovery should go solely to Alexandre Yersin. See Ishigami, *Japanese Text-Book;* and Bibel and Chen, "Diagnosis of Plague."

43. Correspondent, "The International Plague Conference," *China Medical Journal* 25 (1911): 195.

44. Richard P. Strong, ed., *Report of the International Plague Conference Held at Mukden, April 1911* (Manila: Bureau of Printing, 1912).

45. Wu Lien-Teh, *A Treatise on Pneumonic Plague* (Geneva: League of Nations, 1926).

CHAPTER 2: THE MANCHURIAN QUESTION

1. Mo Shen, *Japan in Manchuria: An Analytical Study of Treaties and Documents* (Manila: Grace Trading Co., 1960), 13.

2. Paul H. Clyde, *International Rivalries in Manchuria, 1689–1922* (Columbus: Ohio State University Press, 1928), 13.

3. Rosemary K. I. Quested, *Sino-Russian Relations: A Short History* (Sydney: George Allen and Unwin, 1984), 71–77.

4. Pamela Kyle Crossley, *The Manchus* (Oxford: Blackwell, 1997), 157–165.

5. Ibid. 156–157.

6. Prince Kung (Gong) (11 January 1833–29 May 1898) was a member of the Qing Manchu clan and commonly known at the time as the Sixth Prince. He had strong and cordial ties to Westerners and was recognized for his attempts at modernizing China. With the support of the two dowagers, Kung ruled China until the 1880s, but was demoted after being accused of being rude in front of the dowagers. In the 1890s, after the death of his half-brother, the first Prince Chun, Empress Dowager Cixi asked Prince Kung to return to the court, but he died shortly afterward, unable to effect the needed reforms to save the moribund Qing.

7. Alexander Hosie, *Manchuria: Its People, Resources, and Recent History* (Boston: J. B. Millet, 1910), 191–238.

8. Rosemary K. I. Quested, *"Matey" Imperialists?: The Tsarist Russians in Manchuria, 1895–1917* (Hong Kong: University of Hong Kong, 1982), 91–100.

9. Joshua A. Fogel, "Introduction," in Itō Takeo, *Life Along the South Manchurian Railway: The Memoirs of Itō Takeo*, transl. Joshua A. Fogel (Armonk, N.Y.: M. E. Sharpe, 1988), vii–xxxi.

10. British Foreign Office, *Annual Report, 1909*, British Documents on Foreign Affairs, pt. 1, ser. B, Asia, vol. 9, pp. 136–137.

11. George E. Anderson, "Railway Situation in China," *Special Consular Reports, no.* 48, U.S. Bureau of Manufacturers, Dept. of Commerce and Labor (Washington, D.C.: Government Printing Office, 1911), 9.

12. Ibid., 10–11.

13. Clyde, *International Rivalries*, 34–37.

14. Ibid., 34.

15. Jacques Gernet, *A History of Chinese Civilization*, 2d ed. (Cambridge: Cambridge University Press, 1996), 610–613.

16. Clyde, *International Rivalries*, 57.

17. Michael Hunt, *Frontier Defense and the Open Door: Manchuria in Chinese-American Relations, 1895–1911* (New Haven: Yale University Press, 1973), 11.

18. David Wolff, *To the Harbin Station: The Liberal Alternative in Rus-*

sian Manchuria, 1898-1914 (Stanford: Stanford University Press, 1999), 17. Harbin is a Manchu name meaning "place for drying fishing nets."

19. Ibid., 18-19.

20. Quested, *"Matey" Imperialists?* 100.

21. Wolff, *Harbin Station*, 18.

22. Sergei Witte, *The Memoirs of Count Witte*, trans. and ed. Abraham Yarmolinsky (London: William Heinemann, 1921), 103-104.

23. Clyde, *International Rivalries*, 72.

24. *Parliamentary Papers, 109*, 1899, no.2, quoted in Clyde, *International Rivalries*, 74.

25. Clyde, *International Rivalries*, 79.

26. *The Education of Henry Adams*, vol. 2 (New York: Time, 1964), 175.

27. Frederic Wakeman, Jr., *The Fall of Imperial China* (New York: Free Press, 1975), 220-221.

28. Kanichi Asakawa, "Japan in Manchuria," pt. 1, *Yale Review* (August 1908): 187-188.

29. Adams, *Education*, 225-226.

30. Ibid., 229-230.

31. "Treaty of Portsmouth," full English text in Peter E. Randall, *There Are No Victors Here! A Local Perspective on the Treaty of Portsmouth* (Portsmouth, N.H.: Portsmouth Marine Society, 1985), 95-100.

32. Yukiko Hayase, "The Career of Gotō Shinpei: Japan's Statesman of Research, 1857-1929," Ph.D. diss., Florida State University, 1974, 42-43.

33. Ibid., 12.

34. Tsurumi Yūsuke, *Gotō Shinpei* (An Authorized Biography of Gotō Shinpei) (1937; repr. Tokyo: Sōkei Shobō, 1966), 2:651 [in Japanese]; trans. and quoted by Hayase, "Career of Gotō Shinpei," 107.

35. Itō Takeo, *Life Along the South Manchurian Railway: The Memoirs of Itō Takeo*, transl. Joshua A. Fogel (Armonk, N.Y.: M. E. Sharpe, 1988), 14.

36. Ibid., viii.

37. Hayase, *Gotō Shinpei*, 112-115.

38. Ibid., 125.

39. Yoshihisa Tak Matsusaka, *The Making of Japanese Manchuria, 1904–1932* (Cambridge: Harvard University Asia Center, 2001), 3.

40. Hunt, *Frontier Defense*, 5–11, 246.

41. Roger V. Des Forges, *Hsi-liang and the Chinese National Revolution* (New Haven: Yale University Press, 1973), 188.

42. Quoted in Hunt, *Frontier Defense*, 199.

43. Des Forges, *Hsi-liang*, 153.

44. Hunt, *Frontier Defense*, 259–263.

CHAPTER 3: THE PLAGUE

1. Ivan L. Martinevskii and Henri H. Mollaret, *Epidemiia chumy v Man'chzhurii v 1910–1911 gg.* (Epidemic plague in Manchuria in 1910–1911) (Moscow: Medicina, 1971), 31.

2. There is a discrepancy between dates reported in Russian by Martinevskii and Mollaret and in most other sources. These dates can be reconciled if it is assumed that this Russian source is based on the Julian calendar (OS, Old Style) in use in Russia at the time. These dates differ by thirteen days from the Gregorian calendar (NS, New Style), now in nearly universal use.

3. Roger S. Greene to Secretary of State, "Consular Report No. 111, 12 November 1910," file 158.931/52, RG 59 Washington, D.C.: National Archives (hereafter cited as NA).

4. Martinevskii and Mollaret, *Epidemiia*, 43.

5. Ibid., 33.

6. Greene to Secretary of State, "Consular Report No. 115, 15 December 1910," file 158.931/56, RG 59, NA.

7. Greene to Secretary of State, "Consular Report No. 115, 15 December 1910," file 158.931/52, RG 59, NA.

8. Ibid.

9. Martinevskii and Mollaret, *Epidemiia*, chap. 4.

10. Rosemary K. I. Quested, *"Matey" Imperialists?: The Tsarist Russians in Manchuria, 1895–1917* (Hong Kong: University of Hong Kong, 1982), 100–101.

11. The title *Tao-tai* designated a Qing office that is often translated as "Intendant of Circuit." Under the Qing, the circuit, or "tao," was the

unit of administration just below the province, but more encompassing than the prefectures and counties. It had been established in 627 under the Tang but was abolished as a unit of administration in 1928 as unnecessary. The word *tai* is an honorific meaning "elevated."

12. Roger Sherman Greene was a diplomat, foundation official, medical administrator in China, and a leader in American interest in East Asia. His parents were missionaries in Japan, where Greene received his early education. He received a B.A. (1901) and an M.A. (1902) from Harvard and entered the consular service. He held posts in Brazil, Japan, Siberia, Manchuria, and China. He left a promising diplomatic career to join the Rockefeller Foundation, where his first assignment was with the foundation's commission to survey the medical and public health needs of China. Based on this assessment, the Rockefeller Foundation, through the China Medical Board, established the Peking Union Medical College (PUMC). Greene served as resident director of the board in China, then director of the China Medical Board as well as serving as acting director and director of PUMC until a conflict with John D. Rockefeller (regarding the proper role for religious instruction at PUMC) led to his forced resignation in 1935. See Warren I. Cohen, *The Chinese Connection: Roger S. Greene, Thomas W. Lamont, George E. Sokolsky and American–East Asian Relations* (New York: Columbia University Press, 1978); and "Roger Sherman Greene," *Dictionary of American Biography*, suppl. 4: 1946–1950 (American Council of Learned Societies, 1974).

13. Greene to Secretary of State, "Consular Report No. 112, 12 November 1910," file 158.931/54, RG 59, NA.

14. Greene to Secretary of State, "Consular Report No. 112, 25 November 1910," file 158.931/54, RG 59, NA.

15. Greene to Secretary of State, "Consular Report No. 112, 25 November 1910," file 158.931/54, RG 59, NA. Roger Budberg-Boenninghausen (1867–1926) was "a Baltic German baron and self-taught Sinologist, the only Russian national in Harbin to marry a Chinese woman and to immerse himself in Chinese society." See Mark Gamsa, "The Epidemic of Pneumonic Plague in Manchuria, 1910–1911," *Past and Present* 190 (2006): 147–183.

16. See Quested, *"Matey" Imperialists*, 117. The reference to *Novaya*

Zhizn (New Life) apparently indicates a local publication in Harbin. This is also the name of a well-known Bolshevik daily newspaper printed in Russia between 1904 and 1905 as well as one published by the Mensheviks in 1917 and 1918.

17. H. E. Sly to Sir John Jordan, "Consular Report, 21 December 1910," Public Records Office (hereafter PRO), Foreign Office of the United Kingdom (hereafter FO), 371/1066/269-279a. Sly was acting consul for Great Britain in Harbin, and Jordan was the British ambassador in Peking.

18. Ibid., FO 371/1066/272.

19. Zabolotny had carried out both epidemiological and laboratory studies of plague in the Caucasus, and he held professorships at the St. Petersburg Women's Medical Institute (founded in 1897 as Russia's first medical school for women) and the Odessa State Medical University (founded in 1900 as the medical faculty of Odessa Novorossiyskiy State University). He later served as president of the Ukrainian Academy of Sciences (1927-1928). In 1927 he published his pioneering textbook *Principles of Epidemiology*.

20. Greene provides a list and summary of the articles adopted by the Irkutsk Plague Conference. See enclosure with Greene to Secretary of State, "Consular Report No. 134, 10 March 1911," 158.931/147, RG 59, NA.

21. Dr. Roger Baron Budberg; see Gamsa, "The Epidemic," 179.

22. Greene to Secretary of State, "Consular Report No. 115, 15 December 1910," file 158.931/56, RG 59, NA.

23. Ibid.

24. Ibid.

25. Wu Lien-Teh (pinyin: Wu Liande; Cantonese: Ng Leen-tuck; Hokien: Gnoh Lean-Teik) became known as G. L. Tuck at school in Penang and later at Cambridge.

26. Wu Lien-Teh, *Plague Fighter: The Autobiography of a Modern Chinese Physician* (Cambridge: Hefter, 1959), 667. See also William C. Summers, "Wu Lien-Teh," in *Doctors, Nurses, and Medical Practitioners: A Biobibliographical Sourcebook*, ed. Lois N. Magner (Westport, Conn: Greenwood, 1997). Pei-Yang Medical College was part of Pei-Yang Uni-

versity in Tianjin. Founded in 1895 and modeled after famous Western institutions, the university hoped to modernize China with emphasis on science and technology. Pei-Yang refers to "Northern Ocean," the coastal areas of Zhilin, Liaoning, and Shandong provinces in Northeast China. In 1951 Pei-Yang University was reorganized and renamed Tianjin University.

27. Budberg, described in Gamsa, "The Epidemic," 179.

28. Sly to Jordan, "Consular Report, 3 February 1911," PRO, FO 371/1066/194–198.

29. Greene to Secretary of State, "Consular Report No. 129, 7 February 1911," file 158.931/126, RG 59, NA.

30. Richardson L. Wright and Bassett Digby, *Through Siberia: An Empire in the Making* (New York: McBride, Nast, 1913), 220.

31. Ibid., 221.

32. Greene to Secretary of State, "Consular Report No. 129, 7 February 1911," file 158.931/126, RG 59, NA. See also Sly to Jordan, "Consular Report, 3 February 1911," PRO, FO 371/1066/197–198, which provides a list of names, places of medical education, and affiliations of the twenty physicians. The twenty-five medical students and four sanitary department students remain unnamed.

33. Greene to Secretary of State, "Consular Report No. 130, 14 February 1911," file 158.931/127, RG 59, NA.

34. The detailed account of the initial epidemic in Mukden is from Y. S. Yang, "Notes on the Epidemic of Plague in Mukden," in *Report of the International Plague Conference Held at Mukden, April 1911*, ed. Richard P. Strong (Manila: Bureau of Printing, 1912), 249–253.

35. Alfred J. Costain, *The Life of Dr. Arthur Jackson of Manchuria* (London: Hodder and Stoughton, 1911).

36. Wu, *Plague Fighter,* 37.

37. Hugh Horne to Sir Edward Grey, "Consular Report, 10 January 1911," PRO, FO 371/1066/281–283, and "Consular Report, 17 January 1911," PRO, FO 371/1066/296–298; see also D. K. Kasai, "Summary of Measures Taken Against Plague in South Manchuria," in Strong, *Plague Conference Report,* 253. Horne was British consul in Dairen, and Grey was the British foreign secretary.

38. Kasai, "Summary of Measures," 253–256.

39. Captain von Kayser, quoted in J. C. McNally to Secretary of State, "Quarantine Regulations at Dalny, Manchuria, 7 March 1911," file 158.931/159, RG 59, NA.

40. Kasai, "Summary of Measures," 254.

41. Wu, *Plague Fighter*, 33.

42. Ibid., 29–30.

43. Ibid., 30–31.

44. Wright and Digby, *Through Siberia*, 229.

CHAPTER 4: THE INTERNATIONAL PLAGUE
CONFERENCE AND ITS AFTERMATH

1. Fred D. Fisher to William J. Calhoun, "Dispatch 59, 22 February 1911," contained in Fred D. Fisher to Secretary of State, "Dispatch 62, 25 February 1911," file 158.931/139, RG 59, NA.

2. Fisher to Calhoun, "Dispatch 56, 18 February 1911," contained in Fisher to Secretary of State, "Dispatch 60, 19 February 1911," file 158.931/137, RG 59, NA.

3. In 1902 the external relations of China were reorganized: the *Tsungli Yamen* (Foreign Office) of the Qing government was abolished, and the Department of Foreign Affairs established under the name *Wai wu pu*, literally, "Foreign Function Board."

4. Russian Embassy to Secretary of State, "Memorandum, 19 January 1911," file 158.931/64, RG 59, NA.

5. Wai wu pu to British Legation in Peking, "Telegram, 22 February 1911," Public Records Office, FO371/1066/244.

6. British Foreign Secretary to Count Alexander de Benckendorff, "Note, ca. 25–30 January 1911," PRO, FO 371/1066/259–260.

7. Wai wu pu to British Legation in Peking, "Telegram, 28 January 1911," PRO, FO371/1066/310.

8. Department of State, "Memorandum: Re note from Russian Embassy, Washington to Department of State, 27 January 1911," file 158.931/69, RG 59, NA.

9. Department of State, "Memorandum: Re communication from Yung Kawei to Department of State, 31 January 1911," file 158.931/89a, RG. 59, NA.

10. Department of State to Legations in St. Petersburg and Peking, "Telegram, 9 February 1911," file 158.931/89a, RG 59, NA.

11. Prince Nicholas Koudacheff to Philander C. Knox, "Letter, 18 February 1911," file 158.931/93, RG 59, NA.

12. United States Legation in Peking to Secretary of State, "Telegram, 18 February 1911," file 158.931/103, RG 59, NA.

13. Martin R. Edwards to Secretary of State, "Telegram, 29 January 1911," file 158.931/75, RG 59, NA.

14. Philander C. Knox to Russian Chargé d'Affaires, "Letter, 9 February 1911," file 158.931/89a, RG 59, NA.

15. Paul F. Russel, "Biological and Medical Research at the Bureau of Science, Manila," *Quartly Review of Biology* 10 (1935): 119-153.

16. Richard P. Strong to Secretary of State, "Confidential Report on the International Plague Conference," undated [ca. June 1911], 23, file 158.931/181, RG 59, NA.

17. Minutes, "Re British Delegate for Plague Commission, 11 February 1911," PRO, FO371/1006/332.

18. Strong, "Confidential Report," 24-25.

19. Shibasaburo Kitasato, "Lecture on Plague, Dairen, 17 February 1911 (translation)," PRO, FO371/1067/220-221.

20. Fisher to Secretary of State, "Dispatch, ca. 20 February 1911," file 158.931/138, RG 59, NA.

21. Strong, "Confidential Report," 23.

22. Wai wu pu to British Legation in Peking, "Telegram, 14 February 1911," PRO, FO371/1066/26.

23. Strong, "Confidential Report," 2.

24. Ibid., 19-20.

25. David J. Bibel and T. H. Chen, "Diagnosis of Plague: An Analysis of the Yersin-Kitasato Controversy," *Bacteriological Reviews* 40 (1976): 633-651.

26. Kitasato, quoted in *Manchuria Daily News* (Dairen, 27 March 1911), reported in Carl F. Nathan, *Plague Prevention and Politics in Manchuria, 1910-1911* (Cambridge: East Asian Research Center, Harvard University, 1967), 33-34. Also in Strong, "Confidential Report," 20.

27. Calhoun to Secretary of State, "Telegram, 3 April 1911," file 158.931/149, RG 59, NA. A more expansive description of Kitasato's

vacillation is contained in Calhoun to Secretary of State, "Letter 228, 26 April 1911," file 158.931/173, RG 59, NA.

28. Fisher to Secretary of State, "Dispatch 62, 25 February 1911," file 158.931/139, RG 59, NA.

29. *Sao-Ke Alfred Sze: Reminiscences of His Early Years* (Washington, D.C.: Privately printed, 1962). Sze was junior councilor of the Ministry of Foreign Affairs, Peking, at the time of the plague epidemic in Manchuria. Later he rose through the ranks and in 1921 served as China's minister plenipotentiary in Washington, D.C., a post he held off and on until 1937. He also served as senior adviser of the Chinese delegation that participated in drafting the United Nations Charter in 1945.

30. The Emergency Plague Laboratory from a firm in Berlin was "very compactly packed in five aluminum cases" and cost 6,925 German marks (about $1,650 at pre–World War I conversion of 4.2 marks to the dollar). See Richard P. Strong, "Studies on Pneumonic Plague and Plague Immunization," pt. 1, "Introduction," *Philippine Journal of Science* 7B (1912), 132.

31. Strong, "Confidential Report," 10.

32. Wu, *Plague Fighter,* 45.

33. Ibid.

34. Richard P. Strong, ed., *Report of the International Plague Conference Held at Mukden, April 1911* (Manila: Bureau of Printing, 1912), 4.

35. Ibid., 10–11.

36. Ibid., 10.

37. Ching was professor of Medicine, Therapeutics, and Medical Jurisprudence at the Imperial Medical College in Tientsin, as well as an official of the Fourth Civil Rank and an assistant sub-prefect. See Strong, *Report of the International Plague Conference*, viii.

38. Strong, *Report of the International Plague Conference*, 40.

39. Ibid., 198–199.

40. Strong, "Studies on Pneumonic Plague," 135.

41. Strong, *Report of the International Plague Conference*, 388–397.

42. At the beginning of the conference Dr. Petrie objected to the plan for publication of the final report in Manila and, instead, proposed its publication by Kelly and Walsh, at that time an English newspaper publisher in Shanghai. Since Alfred Sze indicated that the American

offer from Manila had already been accepted, there was no point in discussing it further. The plan was to publish between fifteen hundred and two thousand copies of the report, which was expected to run to six hundred pages. In the final event, it ran to about five hundred pages with two color plates, five black-and-white plates, and six oversize tip-in tables or maps. Sze authorized a limit of six thousand taels or eight thousand pesos to cover the costs of publication. See Strong, *Report of the International Plague Conference*, 30–31. Various currency conversions suggest that this sum was equivalent to about four thousand dollars.

43. Richard P. Strong to Secretary of State, "Letter, 5 June 1911," file 158.931/np, RG 59, NA.

44. Strong to Secretary of State, "Letter, 5 June 1911," 1.

45. Calculation: 1 Kuping (Treasury) tael = 1.2 Troy ounce silver; 1910 silver price = $0.54 per Troy ounce; 1 Kuping tael = 1.2 x 0.54 = $ 0.65.

46. Strong, "Letter, 5 June 1911," 5.

47. John Z. Bowers and Akiko K. Bowers, "Japanese Medicine in Manchuria: The South Manchuria Medical College," *Clio Medica* 12 (1977): 4.

48. Bowers and Bowers, "Japanese Medicine in Manchuria," 4–5.

49. On Mukden Medical College, see D. S. Crawford, "Mukden Medical College (1911–1949): An Outpost of Edinburgh Medicine in Northeast China. Pt. 1: 1882–1917; Building the Foundations and Opening the College," *Journal of the Royal College Physicians of Edinburgh* 36 (2006): 73–79.

50. Carl F. Nathan, "The Acceptance of Western Medicine in Early Twentieth-Century China: The Story of the North Manchurian Plague Prevention Service," in *Medicine and Society in China*, ed. J. Z. Bowers and Elizabeth F. Purcell (New York: Macy Foundation, 1974), 65.

51. Wu, *Plague Fighter*, 450.

52. Nathan, "Acceptance of Western Medicine," 66–68.

53. Wu Lien-Teh, *A Treatise on Pneumonic Plague* (Paris: League of Nations: Health Organization, 1926); also Robert Pollitzer, *Plague* (Geneva: World Health Organization, 1954).

CHAPTER 5: THE PLAGUE'S ORIGIN

1. Pamela Kyle Crossley, *The Manchus* (Cambridge: Blackwell, 1997), 189–205.

2. Alexander Hosie, *Manchuria: Its People, Resources and Recent History* (Boston: J. B. Millet, 1910), 24–25.

3. Crossley, *The Manchus*, 103–104.

4. Ibid. 189–195.

5. Frank Leeming, "Reconstructing Late Ch'ing Fengt'ien," *Modern Asian Studies* 4 (1970): 305–324.

6. Henri Cordier, in *The Catholic Encyclopedia*, vol. 9 (Robert Appleton Co., 1910; online ed., 1999).

7. The Western name for the port of Lüshun became Port Arthur following the use of that place in the second Opium War (August 1860) for repairs of a crippled British frigate under the command of Royal Navy Lieutenant William C. Arthur.

8. Historical Section of the Foreign Office, *Manchuria, No. 69* (London: HMSO, 1920), 24.

9. Ibid.

10. Richardson L. Wright and Bassett Digby, *Through Siberia: An Empire in the Making* (New York: McBridy, Nast, 1913), 216.

11. Wright and Digby, *Through Siberia*, 210–211.

12. Crossley, *The Manchus*, 6–8.

13. For various accounts of the Hong Kong epidemic, see William John Simpson, *A Treatise on Plague Dealing with the Historical, Epidemiological, Clinical, Therapeutic, and Preventive Aspects of the Disease* (Cambridge: The University Press, 1905); William C. Summers, "Congruences in Chinese and Western Medicine from 1830–1911: Smallpox, Plague and Cholera," *Yale Journal of Biology and Medicine*, 67 (1994) 23–32; Carol Ann Benedict, *Bubonic Plague in Nineteenth-Century China* (Stanford: Stanford University Press, 1996); and Mary P. Sutphen, "Not What, but Where: Bubonic Plague and the Reception of Germ Theories in Hong Kong and Calcutta, 1894–1897," *Journal of the History of Medicine and Allied Sciences* 52 (1997): 7–16.

14. Hosie, *Manchuria*, 58–63.

15. See ibid., 61, for a list of his findings.

16. The Amur River (Heilung Jiang) is 1,755 miles long, navigable when not frozen for its entire length, and enters the sea near Vladivostok. Fishing and transportation are the main economic activities associated with the river.

17. For a detailed analysis of the rise of Dalny (Dalian/Dairen) as a Russian port city see Masafumi Asada, "The Chinese Eastern Railway and the Rise of Port Dal'nii (Dalien): 1898–1904" (in Japanese, English abstract) *Slavic Studies* 55 (2008): 183–218.

18. For an extensive history of the development of Dairen under Japanese rule and its importance in the modernization of public health in Manchuria, see Robert J. Perrins, "Doctors, Disease and Development: Engineering Colonial Public Health in Southern Manchuria, 1905–1926," in *Building a Modern Japan: Science, Technology, and Medicine in the Meiji Era and Beyond*, ed. Morris Low (New York: Palgrave Macmillan, 2005).

19. Marco Polo, *The Travels*, transl. and with an introduction by Ronald Latham (Hammondsworth: Penguin, 1958), 98, 330. See also William of Rubruck, "The Journal of Friar William of Rubruck, 1253–1255," in *Contemporaries of Marco Polo*, ed. Manuel Komroff (New York: Dorset, 1989), 66.

20. Anatole S. Loukashkin, "The Tarbagan or the Transbaikalian Marmot and Its Economic Value," *Comptes rendus du XII Congrès International de Zoologie, Lisbonne, 1935*, 2233–2293.

21. Ya. Adya, "Marmot Hunting in Mongolia," in *Holarctic Marmots as a Factor in Biodiversity*, ed. V. Yu. Rumiantsev, A. A. Nikol'skii, and O. V. Brandler, *Abstracts of the Third Conference on Marmots, Cheboksary, Russia, 25–30 August 1997* (Moscow: ABF, 1997), n.p.

22. Loukashkin, "The Tarbagan," 2266–2269.

23. *Encyclopaedia Britannica*, 11th ed., *s.v.* "fur," 354.

24. T. R. V. Parkin, "Fur Dyeing," *Journal of the Society of Dyers and Colourists*, Jubilee Issue (1934): 203–207.

25. Ibid., 204–205. The dyeing of marmot to resemble mink or sable was a complex process. The pelts were first treated with lime and ferrous sulphate, followed by immersion for two hours at 85 degrees Fahrenheit in *p*-phenylene diamine (Ursol D), *p*-aminophenol HCl (Ursol P), pyro-

gallic acid, ammonia, and hydrogen peroxide. After this treatment, additional Ursols were brushed on to give variegated highlights to the furs.

26. Ibid., 205.

27. *Encyclopaedia Britannica*, 11th ed, *s.v.* "fur," 354.

28. Ibid., 348.

29. Ibid., 351.

30. Adya, "Marmot Hunting," n.p.

31. Loukashkin, "The Tarbagan," 2286–2287.

32. Ibid., 2289.

33. Ibid.

34. Frank G. Clemow quoted cases from the Russian literature of 1895 by Biéliavski and Riéshetnikof in "Plague in Siberia and Mongolia and the Tarbagan (*Arcomys bobac*)," *Journal of Tropical Medicine* 3 (1900): 169–174.

35. Ibid., 170.

36. Ibid.

37. N. A. Formozov, A. Yu.Yendukin, and D. I. Bibikov, "Co-adaption des marmottes *(Marmota sibirica)* et des Chasseures de Mongolie," in *Biodiversité chez les marmottes*, ed. M. Le Berre, R. Ramousse, and L. Leguelte (Moscow: International Marmot Network, 1996), 37–42.

38. Ch'uan Shao Ching, "Some Observations on the Origin of the Plague in Manchouli," in *Report of the International Plague Conference Held at Mukden, April 1911*, ed. Richard P. Strong (Manila: Bureau of Printing, 1912), 29.

39. Ch'uan Shao Ching, "Some Observations," 30.

40. Loukashkin, "The Tarbagan," 2288.

41. See, e.g., Mark Harrison, *Disease and the Modern World* (Cambridge: Polity, 2004), 76; and Adrian Wilson, "On the History of Disease-Concepts: The Case of Pleurisy," *History of Science* 38 (2000): 271–319.

42. Samuel K. Cohn, Jr., *The Black Death Transformed: Disease and Culture in Early Renaissnace Europe* (London: Arnold, 2002); David Herlihy, *The Black Death and the Transformation of the West*, ed. S. K. Cohn (Cambridge: Harvard University Press, 1997); Susan Scott and Christo-

pher J. Duncan, *Biology of Plagues: Evidence from Historical Populations* (Cambridge: Cambridge University Press, 2001); and Graham Twigg, *The Black Death: A Biological Reappraisal* (New York: Schocken, 1985).

43. Kirsten I. Bos et al., "A Draft Genome of *Yersinia pestis* from Victims of the Black Death," *Nature* 478 (2011): 506–510; Stephanie Haensch et al., "Distinct Clones of *Yersinia pestis* Caused the Black Death," *PLoS Pathogens* 6 (2010): e1001134; Ole J. Benedictow, *What Disease Was Plague?: On the Controversy over the Microbiological Identity of Plague Epidemics in the Past* (Leiden: Brill, 2010).

44. R. Devignat, "Variétés de l'Espèce *Pasteurella pestis:* Nouvelle Hypothèse," *Bulletin of the World Health Organization* 4 (1951): 247–263.

45. See Dongshen Zhou et al., "Comparative and Evolutionary Genomics of *Yersinia pestis,*" *Microbes and Infection* 6 (2004): 1226–1234; Yanjun Li et al., "Genotyping and Phylogenetic Analysis of *Yersinia pestis* by MLVA: Insights into the Worldwide Expansion of Central Asia Plague Foci," *PLoS ONE* 4 (2009): e6000; and Giovanna Morelli et al., "*Yersinia pestis* Genome Sequencing Identifies Patterns of Global Phylogenetic Diversity," *Nature Genetics* 42 (2010): 1140–1143.

46. Morelli et al., "*Yersinia pestis* Genome Sequencing."

47. Mark Achtman et al., "*Yersinia pestis,* the Cause of Plague, Is a Recently Emerged Clone of *Yersinia pseudotuberculosis,*" *Proceedings of the National Academy of Sciences, U.S.A.* 96 (1999): 14043–14048. The wide range is based on the fact that bv. *antiqua* was involved in the Plague of Justinian, which dates it at least before the sixth century, and molecular clock data, i.e., DNA sequence divergence, estimates its earliest origin about twenty thousand years ago.

48. Zhou et al., "Comparative and Evolutionary Genomics."

49. Achtman et al., "*Yersinia pestis,* the Cause of Plague," and Morelli et al., "*Yersinia pestis* Genome Sequencing"; Benedict, *Bubonic Plague;* Myron Eschenberg, *Plague Ports: The Global Impact of Bubonic Plague, 1894–1901* (New York: New York University Press, 2007); and MacFarlane Burnet and David O. White, *Natural History of Infectious Disease,* 4th ed. (Cambridge: Cambridge University Press, 1972), 230.

50. Yanjun Li et al., "Different Region Analysis for Genotyping *Yersinia pestis* Isolates from China," *PLoS ONE* 3 (2008): e2166.

51. Li et al., "*Yersinia pestis* Isolates from China," 5; Mark Eppinger

et al., "Draft Genome Sequences of Yersinia pestis from Natural Foci of Endemic Plague in China," *Journal of Bacteriology* 191 (2009): 7628–7629.

52. Morelli et al., "*Yersinia pestis* Genome Sequencing," figs. S.2 and S.3.

53. Ibid., fig. S.2.

CHAPTER 6: PLAGUE AND POLITICS

1. Morris Low, "The Japanese Nation in Evolution: W. E. Griffis, Hybridity and Whiteness of the Japanese Race," *History and Anthropology* 11:2–3 (1999): 203–234; see also Sumiko Otsubo, "The Female Body and Eugenic Thought in Meiji Japan," in *Building a Modern Japan: Science, Technology, and Medicine in the Meiji Era and Beyond*, ed. Morris Low (New York: Palgrave Macmillan, 2005).

2. W. W. Rockhill, *China's Intercourse with Korea from the Fifteenth Century to 1895* (London: Luzac, 1905).

3. Baron Speck von Sternburg to Prince von Bulow, "Item XXV.72, 9 September 1907," quoted in E. T. S. Dugdale, *German Diplomatic Documents, 1871–1914*. Vol. 3: *The Growing Antagonism, 1898–1910* (London: Metheun, 1928–1931), 262–264.

4. Harry J. Lamley, "The 1895 Taiwan War of Resistance," in *Taiwan: Studies in Chinese Local History*, ed. Leonard H. D. Gordon (New York: Columbia University Press, 1970), 33.

5. For more on Gotō Shinpei, see Yukiko Hayase, "The Career of Gotō Shinpei: Japan's Statesman of Research, 1857–1929," Florida State University, Ph.D. diss., 1974.

6. Tsurumi Yūsuke, *Gotō Shinpei* (An Authorized Biography of Gotō Shinpei) (1937; repr. Tokyo: Sōkei Shobō, 1966), 2:38 [in Japanese]; trans. and quoted in Hayase, "Career of Gotō Shinpei," 43.

7. Hayase, "Career of Gotō Shinpei," 62.

8. Ibid., 72–74. During the first year of Gotō's tenure, about 80 percent of Taiwan's budget was subsidized by Tokyo. This economic burden was almost completely eliminated by 1905.

9. Tsurumi, *Gotō*, 2:651; transl. and quoted in Hayase, "Career of Gotō Shinpei," 107.

10. South Manchuria Railway Co., *Manchuria: Land of Opportunity* (New York: South Manchuria Railway, 1922).

11. Tsurumi, *Gotō*, 2:815; transl. and quoted in Hayase, "Career of Gotō Shinpei," 124. Also confirmed in Itō Takeo, *Life Along the South Manchurian Railway: The Memoirs of Itō Takeo*, trans. Joshua A. Fogel (Armonk, N.Y.: M. E. Sharpe, 1988), viii.

12. Hayase, "Career of Gotō Shinpei," 122.

13. E. Carlton Baker (1882-19??) was a career diplomat specializing in China. After receiving his B.S. from the University of California in 1905, he was vice-consul and marshal to Foochow, China, in 1906, and from 1907 to 1908 he held the same position at Amoy. In 1909 he was transferred to the Department of State as assistant to the chief of the Division of Far Eastern Affairs and later that year was appointed consul to Antung, China. In August 1911 Baker was appointed consul to Chungking, where he was posted until 1914, when he was appointed consul to Nagasaki. He stayed in Nagasaki only eighteen months before being transferred to Mukden as United States consul.

14. The legality and legitimacy of this treaty is disputed, and it has been rejected in Korea ever since, and later by the Allied Forces occupying Japan after World War II. Korean Emperor Yung-hui refused to sign the treaty as required by Korean law and it was instead signed by Prime Minister Lee Wan-Yong of Korea and Resident General Count Terauchi Masatake of Japan.

15. E. Carlton Baker to W. J. Calhoun, "Dispatch No. 34L, 18 January 1911," file 159/931/107, RG 59, NA, 1.

16. Ibid., 4.

17. Ibid., 10.

18. Ibid., 9.

19. Ibid., 11.

20. Edward H. Zabriskie, *American-Russian Rivalry in the Far East: A Study in Diplomacy and Power Politics, 1895-1914* (Philadelphia: University of Pennsylvania Press, 1946), 148.

21. Boris A. Romanov, *Rossiia v Man'chzhurii, 1892-1906* (Russia in Manchuria, 1892-1906) (Leningrad: Leningradskii vostochnyi institut imeni A. S. Enukidze, 1928); trans. Susan Wilbur Jones (Ann Arbor: American Council of Learned Societies, 1952), 382.

22. Michael H. Hunt, *Frontier Defenses and the Open Door: Manchuria*

in Chinese American Relations, 1895-1911 (New Haven: Yale University Press, 1973), 259-263.

23. B. De Siebert, *Entente Diplomacy and the World: Matrix of the History of Europe, 1909-1914*, ed., arranged, and annotated by George Abel Schreiner (London: George Allen and Unwin, 1921), 24-27.

24. Edward H. Zabriskie, *American-Russian Rivalry*, 175-176.

25. Memo by Minister of Foreign Affairs, 10-23 January 1912, Re: question of Russian recognition of the new Government of Yüan Shih K'ai, in De Siebert, *Entente Diplomacy*, 35.

26. Pamela Kyle Crossley, *The Manchus* (Cambridge, Mass.: Blackwell Publishers, 1997), chap. 7.

27. Kang Chao, *The Economic Development of Manchuria: The Rise of a Frontier Economy* (Ann Arbor: Center for Chinese Studies, University of Michigan, 1983). Chao estimates the population growth in Manchuria as follows: 1898, 6,943,000; 1908, 17,055,000; 1910, 17,942,000; 1914, 19,652,000; and 1930, 31,300,000.

28. Crossley, *The Manchus*, chap. 6.

29. James Reardon-Anderson, *Reluctant Pioneers: China's Expansion Northward, 1644-1937* (Stanford: Stanford University Press, 2005), 83.

30. L. Richard, *Comprehensive Geography of the Chinese Empire and Dependencies*, trans. M. Kennelly, S.J. (Shanghai: T'usewei, 1908), 486, 504-505.

31. Harrison, *Disease*, 2.

32. Hans Zinsser, *Rats, Lice, and History* (Boston: Little, Brown, 1935); and William H. McNeill, *Plagues and Peoples* (Garden City, N.Y.: Anchor Press, 1976).

33. Judith Farquhar, *Knowing Practice: The Clinical Encounter of Chinese Medicine* (Boulder: Westview, 1994).

34. Ruth Rogaski, *Hygienic Modernity: Meanings of Health and Disease in Treaty-Port China* (Berkeley: University of California Press, 2004).

35. Benedict, *Bubonic Plague*; Nathan, *Plague Prevention*; and Rogaski, *Hygienic Modernity*.

36. Warwick Anderson, *Colonial Pathologies: American Tropical Medicine, Race, and Hygiene in the Philippines* (Durham: Duke University Press, 2006), 181-206.

37. Rogaski, *Hygienic Modernity*, 303.

38. See, e.g., David Arnold, *Colonizing the Body: State Medicine and Epidemic Disease in Nineteenth-Century India* (Berkeley: University California Press, 1993).

39. Danny Wynn Ye Kwok, *Scientism in Chinese Thought, 1900–1950* (New Haven: Yale University Press, 1965).

40. The full title of the ranking U.S. diplomat in China was "Envoy Extraordinary and Minister Plenipotentiary to China," a title that was abolished in 1935 and upgraded to "Ambassador Extraordinary and Plenipotentiary."

41. W. J. Calhoun to Secretary of State, "Dispatch No. 228, 26 April 1911," file 158.931/173, RG 59, NA, 9–10.

EPILOGUE

1. Kristen Van Reeth, "Avian and Swine Influenza Viruses: Our Current Understanding of the Zoonotic Risk," *Veterinary Research* 38 (2007): 243–260.

2. K. B. Chua, B. H. Chua, and C. W. Wang, "Anthropogenic Deforestation, El Niño and the Emergence of Nipah Virus in Malaysia," *Malaysian Journal of Pathology* 24 (2002): 15–21.

3. Jonathan L. Heeney, Angus G. Dalgleish, Robin A. Weiss, "Origins of HIV and the Evolution of Resistance to AIDS," *Science* 313 (2006): 462–466.

4. William C. Summers and Sin How Lim, "Epidemiological Concepts with Historical Examples," in *Encyclopedia of Microbiology*, ed. Moselio Schaechter et al., 3rd ed. (New York: Elsevier, 2009).

5. Scott Krauss et al., "Influenza A Viruses of Migrating Wild Aquatic Birds in North America," *Vector-Borne and Zoonotic Diseases* 4 (Fall 2004): 177–189.

6. For two views see N. Howard-Jones, "Origins of International Health Work," *British Medical Journal* 1 (1950): 1032–1037, and David P. Fidler, *International Law and Infectious Diseases* (New York: Oxford University Press, 1999).

7. Karl Taro Greenfeld, *China Syndrome: The True Story of the Twenty-First Century's First Great Epidemic* (New York: HarperCollins, 2006).

8. John M. Barry, *The Great Influenza: The Epic Story of the Deadliest Plague in History* (New York: Penguin, 2004).

9. Diana Crane, *Invisible Colleges: Diffusion of Knowledge in Scientific Communities* (Chicago: University of Chicago Press, 1972).

10. Wu Lien-Teh, *A Treatise on Pneumonic Plague* (Nancy: Berger-Levrault, 1926). Also Wu Lien-Teh et al., *Plague: A Manual for Medical and Public Health Workers* (Shanghai: Weishengshu National Quarantine Service, Shanghai Station, 1936).

11. Giovanni Boccaccio, *Decameron*, trans. and commentator J. G. Nichols (New York: Alfred A. Knopf, 2009).

12. Daniel Defoe, *"A Journal of the Plague Year"*: *Authoritative Text, Backgrounds, Contexts, Criticism*, ed. Paula R. Backscheider (New York: Norton, 1992).

13. Particularly prominent American interests were represented by the railroad tycoon E. H. Harriman and his sometime agent in China, Willard Straight. See Paul H. Clyde, *International Rivalries in Manchuria, 1689–1922*, 2d ed. (Columbus: Ohio State University Press, 1928), 148–200.

Glossary

Aniline dye: A family of chemical dyes based on the nitrogen-containing aniline molecule, invented in Germany in the nineteenth century. These dyes supplanted natural vegetable dyes and became a mainstay of the German chemical industry.

Bacterial toxin: Any substance produced by bacteria that is toxic to its host organism.

Biovar (bv.): Short for "biological variant," a term used to avoid the more specific and precise concept of subspecies.

Chromosomal gene: Gene that resides on the chromosomes of cells as opposed to on the DNA of nonchromosomal cellular elements such as organelles, viruses, and plasmids.

Endemic: A property, usually describing a disease, that is more or less constantly present in a population, as opposed to an epidemic, which is periodic.

Extracellular fluid: Body fluids such as blood plasma, lymph, and tissue fluids that exist outside of cells; in contrast to intracellular fluids, known as protoplasm.

Genomic studies: The examination of the structure of the entire set of genes of an organism (the genome), usually by determination of the sequence of chemical subunits (bases) that make up the DNA and by that sequence encode genetic information.

Hyperimmune serum: Blood serum from an individual who has developed strong immunity through the production of antibodies to a specific microbe, protein, or other immunity-inducing agent.

Lobar pneumonia: An infection and inflammation of the lung tissue that is distributed throughout one or more of the anatomic lobes of the lung.

Lymphatic channels: Fine channels that weave through the tissue to carry body fluids (lymph) through the body outside the blood vessels. They usually lead to the lymph nodes, which function as regional collecting points for the lymph system.

Nipah virus: A normal virus of fruit bats that occasionally can infect pigs, dogs, and sometimes humans with highly lethal consequences. In the first epidemic in Malaysia in 1999 the mortality rate in human cases was 40 percent. The virus was named for the place where the first outbreak occurred.

Plasmid genes: Genes that are encoded in small nonchromosomal DNA molecules that exist as circular, self-replicating structures (plasmids) in the cytoplasm or nucleus of some cells.

Prophylaxis: General term for preventive measures.

Regional lymph nodes: Small globular structures made up of specialized cells of the immune system that are connected together by channels to conduct fluid and immune cells from various regions of the body to the nearby lymph nodes, for example, in the groin and armpit, where bacteria are often trapped and attacked by the immune cells.

Retrograde infection: Any infection that spreads from a peripheral part of the body, for example, one of the limbs, toward the center of the body.

SARS: Acronym for severe acute respiratory syndrome, a condition that was identified in 2003 in Southeast Asia and subsequently associated with infection with a specific agent in the coronavirus family.

Septicemia: Bacterial infection in which the organisms appear in the blood.

Serum/sera: Serum is the liquid part of blood, devoid of the cellular components, the red blood cells, and the white blood cells, which remains after the clotting proteins have been removed by allowing clotting to take place. Sera is the plural form. The serum contains the antibody fraction of blood.

Surface antigen: Any material, usually a protein or sugar molecule, on the surface of a microbe that can elicit an immune response in an infected animal. Often the surface antigens are the targets of immune attack by antibodies in an animal that has been vaccinated or become immune by prior illness.

Treaty of Shimonoseki: The treaty between Japan and China that ended the Sino-Japanese War in 1895, signed in the Japanese city of Shimonoseki. China ceded Taiwan and leased the southern part of Manchuria to Japan, renounced any interest in Korea, and agreed to heavy reparation payments to Japan, among other conditions.

Treaty of Portsmouth: The treaty between Japan and Russia that ended the Russo-Japanese War in 1905, signed in the New Hampshire town of Portsmouth. Russia and Japan both recognized the sovereignty of China in Manchuria, but Japan retained a lease to the southern region as well as certain trading and railroad rights. Treaty negotiations were mediated by the United States, and President Theodore Roosevelt was awarded the Nobel Peace Prize in 1906 for his role in this event.

Vector: Any biological agent, often an arthropod, that can act as an intermediary in transmission of an infectious organism between hosts.

Vector ecology: The totality of conditions that determine the effectiveness of a disease vector, such as habitat, intermediate hosts, natural and acquired resistance, and host biology.

Virulence plasmid: A small, self-replicating extrachromosomal DNA molecule, containing only a few genes, one or more of which convey new properties to the host microbe in which it exists, so as to make the host more virulent or pathogenic.

Index

Page numbers in italic refer to illustrations

INDEX

Great Manchurian Plague (continued)
64, 77, 88, 98, 99, 142, 156, 160; in Port
Arthur, 71, 72, 75, 79; and public health
measures, 15, 71, 129, 138–142, 149–150;
and quarantines, 15, 21, 51, 52–53, 62,
75, 99–100; and railroads, 13–15, 17, 19,
51–52, 53, 54, 59, 61, 62, 63, 66, 67, 69,
71, 78, 80, 100, 129, 139, 141, 146; responses to, 149–150, 162; and Russia,
20–21, 22, 41–42, 51–52, 54–57, *58*,
61–62, 83–84, 106, 159; source of, 22,
53; spread of, 20, 21, 35, 56, 65, 98, 128,
129; and Treaty of Portsmouth, 41–42.
See also International Plague Conference at Mukden
Great Powers: and China, 130, 149; and
Great Manchurian Plague, 1; and
International Plague Conference, 4;
and Manchuria, 110, 130, 138
Greene, Roger S., II, 53, 55–56, 62–63,
65, 66, 172n12, 173n20
Grey, Edward, 83–84, 174n37
Gros (commander of Allied Armies in
China), 30
ground squirrels, 13
Guy de Chauliac, 5

hadj, 157
Haffkine, Paul, 98
Han Chinese, in Manchuria, 47–48, 107,
108, 147–148
Harbin, Manchuria: American consul
in, 53, 55–56, 57, 62–63, 65, 66; Antiplague Bureau, 77; British consul in,
57, 64, 173n17; Chinese administration in, 17, 54, 55, 56, 57, 62–63, 64,
65–66, 68, 75–77, 79, 80, 83, 84, 86,
105, 171–172n11; and Chinese Eastern
Railway, 17, 35, 55, 63, 116, 144, 146;
Chinese investigations of plague in,
19–21, 24–25; corpses accumulated outside hospital near Harbin, *67;* cremation of plague victims in, 75–76, *76;*
Great Manchurian Plague in, 11–12, 14,
19–21, 24–25, 35, 54–57, 59, 61–66, 68,
75–76, 77, 78, 80, 99, 146; and plague
outbreaks, 9; plague workers in, *59;*
population diversity of, 54; quarantines
in, 14, 56, 57, 59, 78, 80, 149; Russian
administration in, 35, 38, 54, 55, 56–57,
58, 59, 61, 62, 66, 68, 78, 79, 80, 83, 84,

88–89, 109, 110, 114, 144, 146, 149, 150;
Russian culture in, 109, 110; as urban
area, 109; wagon carrying dead in, *66;*
Western culture in, 110, 150
Harriman, E. H., 187n13
Harrison, Mark, 148
Hay, John, 39–40, 131
Health Organization of League of
Nations, 105
Heiser, Victor, 86
Hirsch, James G., 166n13
HIV, 153, 154
Holwill (Antung official), 141
Hong Kong, bubonic plague in, 5, 7–8,
13, 112, 128, 129, 159–160
Hong Kong flu, 10
hong merchants, of China, 12
Horne, Hugh, 174n37
Horvath, Dimitri Leonidovic, 144, 145
Hosie, Alexander, 30, 113
host-parasite interactions, 154–155, 156
Hsi Liang (Xiliang): and International
Plague Conference, 81–82, 92, 95, 96,
100; Mukden as official seat of, 67; and
railway expansion, 49–50; and Sino-
Japanese relations, 48–49
human-nonhuman interactions, ecology
of, 154
Hunt, Michael, 35

Ichang fever, 10
Ignatieff (Russian ambassador), 30
Imperial Chinese Railway, 17, 67
Imperial University of Tomsk, Siberia, 61
India, plague outbreaks in, 6
industrialization, in Manchuria, 3–4
influenza, 153, 154, 156, 157, 158, 160
Institute for the Study of Infectious Disease, Tokyo, 88
intermediate hosts, 155
International Plague Conference at Mukden: accounts of, 4; and China, 22–23,
24, 85, 90–92, 103–106, 151; countries
represented, *95;* final report of, 100–
101, 177–178n42; and France, 85; and
geopolitics, 130; and Great Britain, 85,
86, 87–88, 93; and Hsi Liang, 81–82,
92, 95, 96, 100; Interim Report of, 100;
and Japan, 23–24, 85–86, 88, 89, 90–
91, 93, 100, 103–106; key participants
in, *94;* and Kitasato Shibasaburo, 88,

196

Manchouli, Manchuria: Great Manchurian Plague in, 19, 51-53, 54, 56, 61, 97; and marmot fur trade, 110, 124; and plague outbreaks, 124; quarantine in, 52-53, 115; Russia culture in, 109-110; Russians providing medical services in, 51-52, 53, 115; sanitary committee in, 52, 56; as transportation depot, 114
Manchukuo regime: as puppet state, 131, 143; and Sino-Japanese balance of power, 4, 68
Manchu language, 108, 112
Manchuria: bubonic plague outbreaks in, 9-10, 13, 51, 112-113; Chinese administration of, 55; Chinese control of, 15, 26, 47-50, 146-148, 151; compared to American West, 26; culture of, 107, 108-113; foreign consulates in, 18-19; historical role of plague in, 97; infrastructure of, 110-111, 137-138; Japanese takeover of, 1-2, 3, 105, 131, 142-143; 165n2; modernization in, 12, 48, 147-148; political conflicts in, 3, 15; population of, 109, 185n27; Qing dynasty's concept of, 47, 108, 113; railroads in, 15, 16, 17, 27, 30-31, 34-35, 41-42, 44, 47, 108-109, 114, 161; as region of China, 165n2; and Russia, 15, 17, 18, 27, 33-38, 39, 61, 107, 113-115, 130, 143-146, 151-152; and Russo-Japanese War, 3, 142, 146; and Treaty of Portsmouth, 42; and United States, 2-3, 18, 23, 39-42, 50, 130, 138, 139-140, 145. *See also* Great Manchurian Plague (1910-1911); Manchus
Manchurian Plague Prevention Service, 105
Manchurian System, 31
Manchus: assimilation of, 108; and Chinese policies in Manchuria, 47, 48; Chinese racism against, 108, 147; culture of, 107, 108-113; and Korea, 32; Mukden as ancestral home of, 66; and Russia, 28; and Treaty of Nerchinsk, 113; and Tungus ethnolinguistic group, 26
marmots (tarbagans), *117;* and biovars of *Yersinia pestis*, 128; dyeing of fur, 22, 119, 129, 180-181n25; and fur trade, 10, 22, 53, 62, 110, 117, 118-120, 122, 124, 129, 168n40; and Great Manchurian

Plague, 10, 22, 51, 53, 62, 96, 97, 100, 125; hunting of, 10, 51, 53, 110, 117-118, 120-121, 122, 123, 124, 129, 156; and International Plague Conference, 24; names for, 118; and plague outbreaks, 10, 53, 118, 122-123, 125, 129, 156; traditional marmot hunting methods, 120, *121,* 122, 123, 124, 156
Martinevskii, Ivan L., 13, 171n2
Martini (German delegate), 96, 100
medical practitioners, traditional Chinese: and Great Manchurian Plague, 70-71
medical science: and bubonic plague, 7-8; and colonialism, 148; and germ theories of disease, 4, 15, 166n15; and medical history, 4-9, 10, 11, 13, 124-129, 153-154, 166n13; and "uses" of disease, 3
Meiji (emperor of Japan), 3, *42,* 131, 142
Mesny, Girard, 21
microbiology, role of, 3, 88, 168n42
Minami Manshū Igakudō (South Manchuria Medical School), 46
Ming dynasty, 12
Mollaret, Henri H., 13, 171n2
Mongolia and Mongolians: and biovars of *Yersinia pestis*, 128; and Chinese policies in Manchuria, 47, 113; culture of, 108; and fur trade, 118, 119-120; and Manchuria, 26, 35; and marmot hunting, 117, 118, 122, 123; plague outbreaks in, 51, 123; and Russia, 145, 146. *See also* Manchouli, Mongolia
Mongolian marmot (*Marmota sibirica*), 117, *117,* 118, 122
"Mongolian Question," 146
Morelli, Giovanna, 127
Mukden, Manchuria: Chinese administration of, 17, 38, 54, 66-67, 68, 69, 70-71, 78-79, 149; Chinese culture in, 109; Chinese immigration in, 108-109; and Great Manchurian Plague, 19, 22, 54, 63, 66-71, 75, 78-79, 149; house-to-house visitations in, 68-69; and Japanese colonial policy, 116; Japanese establishment of medical school in, 46, 103-104; Manchu culture in, 109; medical missionaries in, 68, 79, 104; quarantines in, 69-70, 79; Russian administration of, 38; and South Manchuria Railway, 17, 46, 48-49, 67, 116,

139; Strong's study of plague in, 90–93; as urban area, 109; Western businessmen in, 68. *See also* International Plague Conference at Mukden
Mukden Medical College, 70, 104
Muravieff Amursky, Nicholas, 28–29, 36

Nathan, Carl F., 11, 12
nationalism, in China, 108, 147
National Quarantine Service, 25, 105
Nian rebellion, 147
Nicholas I (tsar of Russia), 28
Nicholas II (tsar of Russia), 33, 36, 40, 42
Nipah virus, 153, 154
North Africa, plague in, 11
North Manchurian Plague Prevention Service, 24–25, 103, 104–105

Office International d'Hygiène Publique (OIHP), 157, 160
Open Door Policy, 39–40, 47, 50, 131
opium, and Chinese theory of plague's origin, 65
Opium Wars, 29, 30, 179n7
Oriental sore, 10
Oshima (governor-general of the Leased Territory), 81–82

Pan American Health Organization, 160
Pan-Asian movement, 23, 131
paper money, suspected as transmission agent, 65
Pasteur Institute, 8–9
Peiyang Imperial Medical College, 64, 65, 173–174n26
Peking Union Medical College (PUMC), 65, 172n12
Perry, Matthew, 131
Pescadores islands, 32
Petrie, G. F., 87–88, 100, 101, 177n42
Philippines, 150
Pierce, Herbert H. D., 41
plague: bacteriological classification of biovars, 126–129, 182n47; and contagion, 5, 9, 70, 98, 166n15; endemic plague, 13, 53, 124, 128; epochs of, 11; fleas as vector in transmission of, 6, 9, 10, 15, 53, 127; identification of, 4, 6, 8, 23, 64, 122, 166n13, 168n42; manifestations of, 5; meaning of, 4; medical history of, 4–9, 10, 11, 124–129, 153,

166n13; pathology of, 99; and retrospective diagnosis, 125, 126; Zabolotny's study of, 97–98, 173n19. *See also* bubonic plague; Great Manchurian Plague (1910–1911); International Plague Conference at Mukden; pneumonic plague; *Yersinia pestis*
Plague of Athens, 125, 126
Plague of Justinian, 4–5, 10, 11, 125, 126, 182n47
Plague of London, 6, 8, 11, 160, 161
pneumonic plague: causative agent of, 6; Great Manchurian Plague as, 1, 15, 20–21, 22, 51–52, 53, 64, 77, 88, 98, 99, 142, 156, 160; and International Plague Conference, 24; manifestations of, 5; rarity of, 9; Wu Lien-Teh on, 25, 105
poliovirus, 154, 160
Pollitzer, Robert, 105, 160
Polo, Marco, 117–118
Port Arthur (Lüshun), Manchuria: and Great Manchurian Plague, 71, 72, 75, 79; and Japanese culture, 115; population of, 109; and railroads, 30, 34, 36, 41, 71; and Russia, 36, 37, 115; and Russo-Japanese War, 40, 41, 115; Western name, 179n7
Portuguese traders, in China, 12
postcolonial studies, 150
public health measures: and colonialism, 148; and Great Manchurian Plague, 15, 71, 129, 138–142, 149–150; and influenza pandemic (1918), 158; and International Plague Conference, 103; in Japan, 44; in Japanese-controlled regions of Manchuria, 71, 79, 138–143, 149; and modernization, 149; in Russian-controlled regions of Manchuria, 114–115, 144, 146; transnational demands of, 157; and World Bank, 161
Puyi (emperor of China), 102

Qing dynasty: and administration of Harbin, 55, 171–172n11; and administration of Mukden, 68; anti-Qing reformers, 147; and Chinese Revolution, 102; concept of Manchuria, 47, 108, 113; decline of, 3, 4, 147, 149, 169n6; fall of, 50, 146, 151; and foreign affairs, 37–38; and International Plague Conference, 101; investigation of plague in

Qing dynasty (continued)
  Harbin, 19; and Manchu culture, 108,
  112, 113; and modernization in Manchuria, 12, 48, 147; and public health
  measures, 149; and Russia's building
  of Chinese Eastern Railway, 34
quarantines: and bubonic plague in Manchuria, 113; and cholera, 157; in Dairen,
  71–72, 73, 80, 81; and Gotō Shinpei,
  44; and Great Manchurian Plague, 15,
  21, 51, 52–53, 62, 75, 99–100; in Harbin,
  14, 56, 57, 59, 78, 80, 149; in Mukden,
  69–70, 79; Russian enforcement of,
  115; tagging of released persons, 59,
  60
Quested, Rosemary K. I., 144, 167n24

railroads: of China, 31, 47, 49–50; and
  geopolitics, 31, 35, 138; and Great Manchurian Plague, 13–15, 17, 19, 51–52, 53,
  54, 59, 61, 62, 63, 66, 67, 69, 71, 78,
  80, 100, 129, 139, 141, 146; of Japan,
  17, 31, 41, 42–46, 49, 50, 136–137; in
  Manchuria, 15, 16, 17, 27, 30–31, 34–35,
  41–42, 44, 47, 108–109, 114, 161; and
  medical services, 10, 59, 61; and plague
  outbreaks, 5, 9; and plaque control
  efforts, 17; role of, 3; of Russia, 10, 17,
  31, 33, 34–35, 36, 37, 49, 50, 54–55, 114,
  145; and Sino-Japanese relations, 31,
  46, 48–49; and Sino-Russian relations,
  33–37; standards in, 31, 35, 48, 137
rats: and bubonic plague in China, 7, 9;
  and Great Manchurian Plague, 21, 53,
  55, 62, 64, 74, 75; plague associated
  with, 156
Rockefeller, John D., 172n12
Rockefeller Foundation, 55, 172n12
Rockefeller Institute, 86–87
Rogaski, Ruth, 149, 150
Romanov, Boris A., 143
Romanov Empire, 113
Roosevelt, Theodore, 3, 40–41, 42, 134,
  138
Ross, Ronald, 63
Russia: and East Asia, 3, 29, 32; and Great
  Manchurian Plague, 20–21, 22, 41–42,
  51–52, 54–57, 58, 61–62, 83–84, 106,
  159; and International Plague Confer-

ence, 23, 85, 88–89, 90; and Japan, 32,
  37, 40, 133, 137, 143; and Manchuria, 15,
  17, 18, 27, 33–38, 39, 61, 107, 113–115, 130,
  143–146, 151–152; Pacific Rim strategy,
  33; and plague outbreaks, 9, 10, 13–14,
  167n24; railroads of, 10, 17, 31, 33, 34–
  35, 36, 37, 49, 50, 54–55, 114, 145. *See
  also* Russo-Japanese War (1904–1905);
  Sino-Russian relations
Russian Sanitary Department, 14
Russo-Japanese War (1904–1905): and
  Japanese acquisition of Dairen, 109,
  115; and Japanese railroads in Manchuria, 31, 44, 67, 136, 143; and Manchuria, 3, 142–143, 146; Theodore
  Roosevelt's mediation of, 40–41;
  and spheres of influence, 143

Sakhalin Island, 29, 41
San Francisco epidemic (1900), 13
Sanitary Board, 112–113
Sazonov, Sergi, 145, 146
schistosomiasis, 155
Scientific Research Institute, Peking, 101
scientism, 151
Second Opium War, 30, 179n7
severe acute respiratory syndrome
  (SARS), 153, 158, 160
Shah-Hsi Temple, 69
Shibayama Gorosaku, 90, 93, 96
Siberia, 85
Siberian Railway Committee, 33
Simond, Paul-Louis, 8–9
Simpson, W. J., 87
Sino-Japanese Agreement (1905), 48–49
Sino-Japanese relations: and adminis-
  tration of Dairen, 81–82; and Antung,
  138–143; and Chinese sovereignty, 103,
  149; and Dairen, 81–82; and Inter-
  national Plague Conference, 88; and
  Korea, 32, 131–132, 133, 134; and Man-
  chukuo regime, 4, 68; and Manchuria,
  47, 48, 147, 148; and railroads, 31, 46,
  48–49; and sacking of Peking, 38; and
  Treaty of Shimonoseki, 32
Sino-Japanese War (1894–1895): and
  China's war reparations, 3; and Gotō,
  44; and Korea, 32, 132–133; and Manchuria, 32, 142–143; and Russia, 33;

and Sino-Japanese relations, 23; and
Taiwan, 43, 133, 135, 136
Sino-Russian relations: and administration of Harbin, 54–57, 59, 61, 62–63,
79, 80, 84, 144; and Chinese sovereignty, 57, 80, 85; and Germany, 36;
and international intervention in Manchuria, 82, 83, 84–85; and Manchuria,
47, 48; and Muravieff, 28–30, 36; and
railroads, 33–37; and sacking of Peking,
38; and secret accord (1896), 34; and
Treaty of Nerchinsk, 27–28; and
Treaty of Peking, 30
Sly, H. É., 57, 64, 173n17
smallpox virus, 154, 156–157, 158
South Asia, plague outbreaks in, 11
Southeast Asia, plague outbreaks in, 11
South Manchuria Medical College, 103,
104
South Manchuria Railway: and Dairen,
17, 45, 71–72, 79, 81; hospitals maintained by, 46; and International Plague
Conference, 91, 93; and Japanese colo-
nial policy, 31, 44–45, 114, 116, 136–
138, 148; and Japanese influence, 115;
Japanese personnel of, 86; Kitasato's
inspection tour of, 88; and medical
school in Mukden, 46, 103; Mukden-
Antung line, 17, 46, 48–49, 67, 116, 139;
research department of, 45, 137–138;
and Treaty of Portsmouth, 41, 44; and
Western culture, 110
Soviet Union, 157–158. *See also* Russia
Spain, and Japan, 32
spongiform encephalopathies, 162
squirrels, 13
Stanley, Arthur, 89, 100, 101
Sternburg, Speck von, 134
Stitt, Edward R., 86
Straight, William, 50, 187n13
Strong, Richard P.: and International
Plague Conference, 22, 24, 87, 88–93,
99, 100, 101; and Scientific Research
Institute in Peking, 101–102
Sun Yat-sen, 103
Sutton, Willie, 159
Sydenham, Thomas, 160
Sze, Sao-Ke Alfred, 92, 96, 100, 101–103,
177n29, 177–178n42

Taiping rebellion, 29, 147
Taiwan, and Japan, 32, 42–43, 133, 135–
136, 137, 183n8
Tao-tai, 55, 56, 57, 62, 92, 171–172n11
tarbagans. *See* marmots
Teague, Oscar, 22, 89–90, 92, 96, 100,
101–102
technology: and disease, 3; and Japan,
131; and modernization, 174n26; and
spread of Great Manchurian Plague,
129
Terauchi Masatake, 184n14
Thucydides, 126
timber resources in Manchuria, 18, 26,
46, 139
Tokyo Imperial University, 104
trade: in China, 12, 17; in Korea, 132; and
Manchuria, 27, 44, 47, 100, 110, 116.
See also fur trade
transportation systems: and Amur River,
114, 180n16; and Manchuria, 27; and
plague outbreaks, 5. *See also* railroads
Trans-Siberian Railway, 17, 33, 36, 40, 41
Treaty of Nerchinsk (1689), 27–28, 113
Treaty of Peking (1860), 30
Treaty of Portsmouth (1905): and Chi-
nese sovereignty, 46; and division of
railways, 15, 16, 17, 41, 44; French post-
card depicting, 42; and Japanese colo-
nialism, 48; political cartoon, 43; and
Theodore Roosevelt, 3, 41; terms of,
41–42, 50; and troops for railroad
administration, 15, 23
Treaty of Shimonoseki (1895), 32, 43, 133
Treaty of Tientsin (1858), 30
treaty ports, of China, 12
Triple Intervention, 32, 133
Truppel (governor), 72
Tsang Woo Huan, 95
tuberculosis, 153, 155
Tuck, G. L. *See* Wu Lien-Teh (Wu
Liande)

United Nations, 157, 158
United States: and China, 38, 49–50,
101–102, 106; and Cold War, 157–158;
Harbin consul, 53, 55–56, 57, 62–63, 65,
66; and International Plague Conference, 24, 85, 86–91; and Japan, 80–81,